THE WELL-ROUNDED
Pregnancy Cookbook

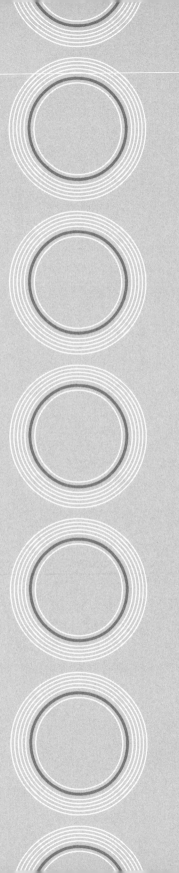

THE WELL-ROUNDED
Pregnancy Cookbook

Give Your Baby a Healthy Start with **100 RECIPES**
That Adapt to Fit How You Feel

Karen Gurwitz with Jen Hoy

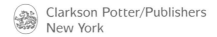
Clarkson Potter/Publishers
New York

Copyright © 2007 by Karen Gurwitz

All rights reserved.
Published in the United States by Clarkson
Potter/Publishers, an imprint of the Crown Publishing
Group, a division of Random House, Inc., New York.
www.crownpublishing.com
www.clarksonpotter.com

Clarkson N. Potter is a trademark and Potter and colophon
are registered trademarks of Random House, Inc.

Recipes on pages 57, 60, 80, 87, 101, 112, 114, 118, 120, 122,
128, 184, 186, and 206 printed with permission from Jen Hoy.

Library of Congress Cataloging-in-Publication Data
Gurwitz, Karen.
    The well-rounded pregnancy cookbook : give your baby
a healthy start with 100 recipes that adapt to fit how you feel
/ Karen Gurwitz with Jen Hoy.
        p.   cm.
Includes index.
1. Pregnancy—Nutritional aspects.   2. Mothers—Nutrition.
3. Cookery.   4. Menus.   I. Hoy, Jen.   II. Title.
RG559.G87   2007
641.5'6319—dc22   2007006071

ISBN 978-0-307-35181-4

Printed in the United States of America

Design by Danielle Deschenes

10   9   8   7   6   5   4

First Edition

For Dori and our angels
Nika, Sophie, and Ethan

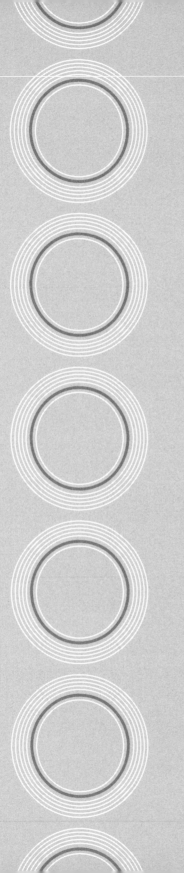

⌘ Contents

Preface

When Karen asked me to write the foreword to this book, she presumably was think-ing of me as a nutrition expert. But when I accepted, I was thinking of myself as a husband and a dad. My wife, Catherine, and I have five children. Pregnancy has been a big part of our lives, and as for us all, wonderful, challenging, episodically torment-ing, and of course, life changing.

In preventive medicine, we refer to the occasional opportunities we have to influence people in a way that will nurture their health as "teachable moments." Unfortunately, all too often, the teachable moment comes later than it should—for example, right after a heart attack. All of a sudden, someone who could have avoided heart disease in the first place is "born again" with a zeal for healthy living. My col-leagues and I are happy to do all we can with these opportunities, so we at least help that person avoid even more health trouble down the line. But these after-the-fact opportunities to pursue health don't make us nearly as happy as we would be to see health nurtured as a cherished priority from birth!

And that's where Karen comes in. She knows that pregnancy is the greatest of all "teachable moments"—an opportunity, an invitation, and perhaps even an obliga-tion, to indulge in the pursuit of your own health, while building the foundation of lifelong health for your baby. There could scarcely be a more important investment, nor a greater potential return. And as you confront the unique challenges and rich promise of pregnancy, you could not hope for a better investment counselor than Karen.

For starters, she is a wise, thoughtful, intelligent, caring, and sensitive person. We could all do with occasional advice from someone with those credentials! But of course, she is so much more. Karen is a mother of three and thus has the intimate understanding of all the challenges of pregnancy that can only come from firsthand experience.

After the birth of her third child, she found herself balancing taking care of two toddlers, a newborn, and her fledgling business while not losing sight of her own needs and desires. While for many of us that might have been a daunting set of tasks, for Karen it was, to borrow from my friends at *O* magazine, an "aha moment." Karen has found the way to nurture herself and her family, and to help you do the same, not along the unrealistic path of least resistance, but by navigating around the challenges of the real world, just like the rest of us.

The dietary guidance Karen offers here is as practical as it is prudent. Karen commits herself to high standards of healthful nutrition, while avoiding the danger of making perfect the enemy of good. You not only should do as she advises—you truly can!

As for the culinary merits of Karen's guidance, they are scarcely in question. Before this book was ever a twinkle in a publisher's eye, Karen was successfully running her wonderfully innovative catering company, Mothers & Menus. This lady not only knows how to nurture health and pregnancy as they deserve—she really knows how to cook!

I love that this book is about healthful nutrition, but not only that. It's about caring for yourself, your baby, and your family in a wholesome, holistic way. It's about finding pleasure in the pursuit of health, and health in the pursuit of pleasure. It's about you, and also about your connections to the people who surround you. And, of course, it's about a vital, healthful, joyful start in life for your baby.

Pregnancy is an indelible passage, a defining time in the lives of all those touched by it. Karen will guide you through that passage toward both greater joy and better health, for you and your baby. That is an undeniably well-rounded destination, and this book offers a well-blazed trail right to it. I encourage you to follow it.

David L. Katz, M.D.
Director, Yale Prevention Research Center
Associate Director, Nutrition Science,
   Rudd Center for Food Policy & Obesity, Yale University
Associate Professor, Adjunct, Public Health,
   Yale University School of Medicine
Medical Contributor, ABC News
Nutrition Columnist, *O, the Oprah Magazine*
www.davidkatzmd.com

Foreword

As an obstetrician who has delivered more than a thousand babies, I am keenly aware of the importance and the impact of healthy eating during pregnancy. There is simply no way around it—a healthy diet leads to an easier pregnancy and delivery, a quicker recovery, and a healthier baby.

But as a working mother of two, I also know how challenging it can be to eat well when you are too busy, too tired, or, quite frankly, just not in the mood to cook a healthy meal. The trip to the grocery store alone, to pick up fruits and vegetables and decipher food labels, can be time consuming.

This is where *The Well-Rounded Pregnancy Cookbook* comes in, with realistic ways to address these issues. In it, Karen discusses the importance of healthful eating before, during, and after pregnancy, and how her own personal struggles with weight helped her to embrace a healthy diet and happy medium. Her honesty is compelling—when reading her words you feel as if you were speaking to an old friend. And, as an old friend would do, she offers helpful advice, encouraging you to acknowledge and embrace your moods and offering you recipe adaptations to keep you on track. Her expertise comes not as a doctor, a chef, or a nutritionist, but rather as a peer—a fellow mom who learned about healthy eating along the way and wants to share her experiences with you.

That said, Karen is not exactly a novice when it comes to the subject of eating healthfully during pregnancy. She is the founder of Mothers & Menus, an organic-meal delivery service for expectant and new moms. She has served hundreds of families fresh, balanced, tasty meals daily. I love that this book incorporates the real stories of real women—Mothers & Menus clients—who cook delicious healthy meals while pregnant or, even more remarkably, with toddlers in their kitchens. I wish I had had this service when I was a new mother!

There are so many important issues to deal with during pregnancy. With the suggestions that Karen offers in her cookbook, she helps take the stress out of healthy eating and makes it an enjoyable experience, all while being realistic about the ideal. For example, she lets you know that organic may be best, but shares that everything is not completely organic in her home kitchen. Karen offers suggestions for incorporating organic foods into your lifestyle with a personal understanding of what it takes to make changes to eating habits. This is similar to how I approach ideal situations with my own patients. Although I would love to see every woman reach her ideal weight before she becomes pregnant, I know that this is not always realistic, so I advocate a balanced diet and exercise during pregnancy to moderate weight gain for the health of mom- and baby-to-be.

Most of all, I appreciate how Karen emphasizes the importance of taking care of yourself. A healthy diet prior to pregnancy, during pregnancy, and in the early years of your child's life is a wonderful gift to yourself as well as your child. So take care of yourself, eat well, and have a happy and healthy pregnancy!

Laura E. Riley, M.D., OB/GYN

Medical Director, Labor and Delivery,
    Massachusetts General Hospital
Assistant Professor, Obstetrics, Gynecology,
    and Reproductive Medicine, Harvard Medical School
Author of *You and Your Baby: Pregnancy* and
    You and Your Baby: Healthy Eating During Pregnancy

Introduction *The Journey*

For as long as I can remember, I was a nurturer—babysitting, making dinner, offering the shoulder of choice for a friend in need. As I got older, this characteristic came in quite handy. Being responsible, efficient, and an excellent listener allowed me to climb the corporate ladder and become a young marketing executive in technology. Everyone knew I could be counted on to get the job done. As busy as I was, there was always room for more on my plate, and so more got piled on. Taking care of others came so naturally to me. When I was burnt out, upset, or angry, I used food to keep me going, push down my feelings, and give myself a "treat." It was all about doing, doing, doing. It wasn't until I got pregnant that I slowed down enough to see how I was taking care of myself. I wasn't.

Something about caring for a developing human being allowed me to shift my priorities and put myself at the top of the list—not for me, but for the growing baby within. Being pregnant gave me permission to start asking for the things I needed and to look at my eating in a new light. In my fast-paced life I had gotten used to skipping meals, loading up in the evenings, dieting for a few days, and then overeating on others. I didn't give much thought to what I was putting into my body, as long as I looked okay.

Being pregnant allowed me to see food in a new light: as nourishing, life-giving, and energizing, with the power to be good for me and good for my baby. As my perspective changed, so did my eating. I moved away from highly processed junk and diet food and turned to whole, natural foods—real food, food as close as possible to its source, like fruits, vegetables, beans, and whole grains. I ate regular meals and snacks, and I felt great.

My first child was born in February 2001. I was high on adrenaline for the first few days and did not think about anything but the amazing little creature in front of me. Four weeks later, though, I still felt quite round, and my immediate impulse was to go on a diet. But as a new mother, my thoughts turned to my baby. What if I did not make enough milk to nourish her? If I cut down on my calories, would that cut down on hers? So I stuck to my plan of eating whole foods, chopping up salads, preparing dinners, bagging my snacks to go, and calculating my nutritional intake.

After six weeks, I was exhausted. I was spending so much time and energy worrying about food, carefully crafting nutritious meals that would be good for me and my baby. I wanted to call someone who would tell me what to eat, make it, and bring it to me every day! I went online and made some calls, but could not find what I wanted. I figured it was just me, but as I joined new mothers' groups, I heard other moms say the same thing. They weren't clear on what was good for them and their babies, and if and when they figured it out, they just couldn't find the time or the energy to plan their meals. I held focus groups in my home, interviewed mom after mom, and eventually created an organic-meal delivery service for expectant and new mothers. I called it Mothers & Menus, because every mother needs her own menu. When I met Jen Hoy, a chef, nutritionist, and intuitive healer, whose passion is helping women nourish themselves, I knew I had struck gold.

Having tried out almost every diet ever marketed, I had come to terms with the fact that there are no shortcuts. The best way to maintain a healthy eating regime is to do just that: eat a balanced diet and make room for cravings with moderation. So I set out to build the Mothers & Menus program that way. The menus are based on whole foods, which are easier to digest and alleviate fatigue and mood swings, common side effects of pregnancy (and motherhood). They are on the opposite ends of the spectrum from junk food, which not only has little nutritive value but can also contain harmful additives, be difficult to digest, and make you tired. As part of our commitment to mothers and their babies, the food is mostly organic. (If you do not generally eat organic foods, pregnancy is a great time to incorporate some key ingredients into your diet; more about this is in Chapter 2.) The final component of our menus is customization. We adapt each mother's menu to her specific needs, based on her pregnancy, lifestyle, and cravings. Jen sticks to the optimal health plan, while I keep the mom's cravings and comfort foods in mind. Then we get to work. "Karen, that mom needs some more miso and kale." "But, Jen, what she wants is some pasta and a cupcake." Back and forth we go, finally compromising on some miso and a salad for lunch, a cupcake for a snack, and some pasta with kale for dinner.

This is what makes Mothers & Menus different from any other meal delivery service available. It is also what makes this cookbook unique. We selected the most sought-after recipes in our experience. More important, you'll find variations for nearly every recipe, so that you can tune in to your own needs and choose one recipe that most suits your mood.

I am happy to say that I've done the heavy lifting for you: here are 100 simple, delicious recipes that are good for you and good for your growing baby. The guesswork is gone, and the recipes make it all so easy. Now it is up to you to tap into your own intuition, recognize what your body needs, and feed it accordingly. Pregnancy is a unique opportunity to tune out distracting voices and focus on yourself. After all, it's your body, your baby, your pregnancy, and your mood. Use this cookbook as a tool to support, nurture, and nourish you wherever you are on your journey of motherhood.

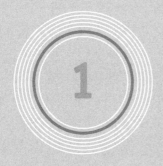

Taking Care of You

By the time I graduated from high school, I could relay the calories in any food faster than my multiplication tables. As I grew older, I played with different extremes, from liquid diets to a vegan regime. Overweight for most of my life, I was up for anything. As I prepared my body for pregnancy, however, I realized that my yo-yo dieting was not going to work. I knew I had to look for something that would nurture my body and ultimately nourish my baby within. I found my balance in the form of whole foods: natural, minimally processed foods, closest to their original form. This felt good to me. It was how I ate when I was pregnant with each of my children, how I got back to my prepregnancy weight, and how I continue to eat today.

Early in her pregnancy, my best friend, Lilly, asked me what she should be eating. She had always been thin and while she was not concerned that eating chocolate ice cream would leave her heavier, she was worried that it would not be nourishing her baby. When I founded Mothers & Menus, an organic-meal delivery service for expectant and new moms, I began to see that regardless of how women had regarded food throughout their lives, being pregnant made them stop and take a look at what they were eating, and how it would nurture their babies. Athletes wondered about adapting their eating to their decreased, but still active, exercise levels; overweight women were looking to keep their weight gain within recommended limits for their babies and their own health; slimmer clients were concerned about eating enough to have a healthy-sized baby. But beyond weight gain, they were all primarily concerned about getting the right nutrients. No matter where they were starting from, the core was the same. They all wanted to provide their babies with the first thing they could give: a healthy start.

I once read that 80 percent of women revamp their diets when they get pregnant. I can't substantiate that claim, but it sure makes sense to me. What better time to make a change, when what you eat can have a direct impact on your baby's health? And so the mothers-to-be adapt their eating habits, incorporating greens, drinking milk, and taking multivitamins. But pregnancy has a way of throwing you curve

PUT ON YOUR OXYGEN MASK FIRST

Before having kids, I caught up on my reading while the flight attendants performed their demonstrations. But as a new mom, I became attentive to their message: "If you are traveling with a child, put on your oxygen mask first, and then attend to the child." This has become my mantra in life. If I am not caring for myself, I cannot care for my kids in the best way possible. Ideally, this would involve a life of personal assistants for weekly massages, strength training, and manicures. But let's start with the basics. Making sure that you are well fed, well rested, and feeling good is the best way to allow yourself to tap into your motherly instincts and best care for your child. That is what *The Well-Rounded Pregnancy Cookbook* sets out to help you do.

balls along the way—nausea, cravings, and hormonal changes can leave women feeling confused and sabotaged. One Mothers & Menus client, Charis San-Antonio Cooper, a longtime vegetarian, suddenly found herself wanting beef in the worst way when she became pregnant. At first, she ignored her cravings, thinking they would pass, but a few months into her pregnancy, she found the desire was too strong to overcome. "I couldn't believe how ravenous I was for meat! The smell of a good steak got me going. It was nuts!" When Lauren Slayton, a registered dietician and the founder of New York City–based Foodtrainers nutritional counseling center, became pregnant with her second child, she found herself repelled by greens. She wanted no salads, spinach, or broccoli—the staples of her usual regime. Instead she craved salty fried foods around the clock, while counseling her clients to eat them in moderation. "It was a little strange for me at first, but because it was the only thing that my body would take, I accepted it as natural. My husband's reaction was much stronger; he kept asking, 'Are you ever coming back?'"

As your body starts changing and you begin to tune in to your needs, you may be surprised by what you feel, what you want, what you need, because it is so different than who you know yourself to be. But parenting is a great time to give yourself room to grow. Like your body, let your emotions and mind expand. Try out your intuition, nurture your body, honor your cravings, and if compelled to do so, try a new food you swore you never would eat. Charis's ventures into meat worked out so well for her, she completely gave up her vegetarian lifestyle when Max was born, and does not miss it. Give yourself permission to break your own rules and trust that your budding inner mothering instincts will guide you the right way.

Cooking on Your Terms

We know that our meals are nutritious and our clients tell us they are delicious, but for this cookbook, we wanted to choose recipes that would also be easy to take on at home. This meant leaving out some Mothers & Menus favorites, like the raved-about Red Bean, Bhutanese Rice, and Sweet Potato Veggie Burger, which requires fifteen ingredients and over an hour of chopping to prepare. It also meant having real people with real lives try out the recipes and give us their feedback. Look for their stories in "Real World" sidebars. As a result, the recipes are foolproof.

What really sets this cookbook apart from any other book aimed at pregnant or nursing women, however, is that nearly every recipe can be adapted to fit how you feel. Three recipe variations—Feeling Green, Feeling Food, and Feeling Full—help you respond to those pregnancy curveballs, such as morning sickness and cravings, and change a recipe accordingly. Here's how it works: The main recipes provided are based on an optimal eating plan, one that will help you feel grounded and balanced. If you can use these recipes 70 percent of the time, you will be following a nutritionally favorable eating plan that is good for you and your baby.

FEELING GREEN: Unfortunately, almost 56 percent of women experience nausea with their pregnancies—and this differs from pregnancy to pregnancy for individual women. Anyone who has had this sensation knows that calling it "morning sickness" is an ironic nomenclature made up by someone who has never felt green all day long or been hit by the nausea waves when she least expected them. This awful feeling can be doubly cruel for a woman who is having trouble gaining the recommended amount of weight at any time during her pregnancy, in which case mealtimes may become even more stressful. Feeling Green provides you with recipe suggestions to help you make it through the meal, day, trimester, or (bless you) the whole nine months. Too green to get into the kitchen? Pass this book on to your spouse, mom, or friend and mumble something about what you want in order to point them in the right direction.

FEELING FOOD: Feeling Food is about honoring your cravings, specifically the ones that sound something like, "Hmmm, I sure feel like a cheeseburger right now." You may know that a cheeseburger is not the most optimal meal, but as you continue to think about it (or try not to), the desire intensifies. Pregnancy is notorious for triggering cravings, many of which are signals from your body for a nutrient you may need. Usually, however, the craving shows up as some form of a childhood meal or comfort food. Feeling Food is a play in balance, offering you a recipe variation that will satisfy your craving while providing you with the nutrients you need to keep on track and stay healthy.

FEELING FULL: Whether you are trying to conceive, are already pregnant, or are a new mom, you are bound to hit a day when you feel extra full, extra bloated, or extra round and want to eat a little lighter. Let me emphasize that conception, pregnancy, and nursing are *not* times for dieting. But there are days when you need to incorporate additional nutrients and hold off on empty calories. If your doctor has warned you of rapid weight gain during the pregnancy, if you have finished nursing and are ready to shed some pounds, or if you just want to take your already healthy eating up another notch, Feeling Full is the recipe variation to use.

Beyond the recipes, I've stashed some other tips and hints throughout the book. Look for "Express" guidelines to help speed things up. While I love the thought of creating a fresh vegetable broth as a basis for all of my soups, I gladly give in to store-bought organic broth as needed. "Legend has it . . ." is a taste of the history of the meal or an ingredient. Read through these little notes as you stir, steam, and fold. Some are informational, others just entertaining tidbits, balancing the need-to-know with a little bit of heritage.

In the end, it is all about balance—finding a balance that works for you, so that you can be there for yourself and for your family.

2

❖ Feeding Your Body

Two months ago, I got a long-awaited call from my college roommate, Yael. After two long years of trying, she is pregnant with twins. Hooray! We laugh and cry and cheer and then get down to business. Yael wants to go over her eating with me because she knows that she needs to get a certain amount of calories to nourish her babies. Normally, this would not be a concern for her. In our dorm, Yael was famous for putting away a whole pizza without gaining a pound, finishing off her plate and yours, and always being up for dessert. But for the first time in her life, Yael is not hungry.

Pregnancy is an amazing time for so many reasons, not the least of which are the physical and emotional changes that you experience in your body. It is not uncommon to go from being someone who is used to eating frequently to experiencing a decrease in hunger, and conversely, to go from being a mild grazer to feeling downright ravenous. The trick, as always, is to find the balance that will take care of your needs while also caring for your baby.

First, the facts. The American Dietetic Association maintains that the appropriate weight gain for women during pregnancy is as follows: 25 to 35 pounds for a woman of normal weight, 28 to 40 pounds for an underweight woman, and 15 to 25 pounds for an overweight one. For a mother of twins with normal weight, the number rises to 35 to 45 pounds, and for triplets, 50 to 70 pounds. In my experience, the weight gain changes from person to person and sometimes from pregnancy to pregnancy. I gained 40 pounds with Nika, 18 pounds with Sophie, and over 65 pounds with Ethan. Each experience was completely different and unique to where I was in my life at the time. Among my clients I see some of everything. Many people fall within the recommended range, but others do not.

How does recommended weight gain translate into calories? When you are pregnant, you need 300 additional calories per day during your second and third trimesters. If you are pregnant with twins, this number is 500—that means, 300 to 500 calories in addition to whatever the normal and healthy intake is for you based on your height and activity levels. (Statistically, the number is 1,831 calories for the average American woman who is *not* pregnant.) When you are nursing, you need to add 500 calories for a single baby and 800 to 1,000 for twins. The average American woman nursing twins should therefore consume up to 2,831 calories a day.

Since our society is preoccupied by counting calories and keeping them low, just thinking about these numbers can get you concerned. But there are other issues to factor in: foods to avoid during pregnancy; cravings for the exact foods you should be avoiding; possible nausea; and a long list of nutrients, vitamins, and minerals that you need to incorporate into your daily diet.

So hang on. Let's try something else. Let's look at how we can incorporate all the foods that will nourish and nurture you and your baby while you are pregnant (which would also nourish and nurture you when you are not).

Eat Whole Foods

Whole foods are minimally processed and as close to their natural form as possible. These are real foods: natural foods like fruits, vegetables, and real cheese, instead of processed; whole wheat flour instead of refined white flour. They contain valuable nutrients, and if you stick to whole foods, you do not have to worry about potentially harmful additives. Whole foods are especially helpful during and right after pregnancy because they contain fiber and water, which make it easier for your body to process these foods, thus alleviating the fatigue that comes with difficult digestion. The fiber in whole foods is filling and brings nutrients to your body in their most effective form. Eating a whole foods–based diet leaves you feeling grounded and balanced. Don't get me wrong: there is *nothing* wrong with eating processed foods. But if you can make whole foods the staple of your diet and refined foods a once-in-a-while kind of thing, your body will take all the vitamins, minerals, and proteins that it needs from the whole foods and balance itself out.

Enjoy Balanced Meals

Whole, unrefined foods are fabulous, but you need a daily mix of fresh fruits and vegetables, "good" carbohydrates, proteins, and fats.

1. *Fresh fruits and vegetables:* Whenever you reach for a snack or start preparing your meal, look for a way to work in a fruit or a vegetable. When choosing fruits and vegetables, look for an array of color to provide a range of vitamins and minerals. And hold a special place in your heart for all things leafy and green. Integrating a dark, leafy green vegetable (such as kale, spinach, dandelion, bitter greens, or broccoli) into your daily diet will add crucial fiber, vitamins, minerals, and chlorophyll, a powerful antioxidant.

2. *Carbohydrates:* It is true that you need carbohydrates as part of a healthy, balanced diet. It is also true that some carbohydrates can make you feel sluggish and

cause weight gain. Figuring out the differences between various kinds of carbo-hydrates can be confusing.

Time to bring in some science to sort all of this out: A simple carbohydrate is comprised of small molecules of sugar, which are quickly and readily absorbed into your system. It does not provide sustained energy. Cakes, cookies, white breads, and pastas are all examples of foods high in simple carbohydrates. They give a quick sugar high followed by a low that may leave you tired or irritable and looking for another fix. Complex carbohydrates, such as whole grains, are made up of longer molecular strands of simple sugars, which include fiber and starches. Because it takes longer for your body to digest these sugars, they are more satisfying than simple sugars and provide you with sustained energy.

There's a little more to this story: Recent research shows that the effect that food has when entering your bloodstream also determines whether a carbohy-drate is good or bad for you. So, while a regular baked potato is a complex car-bohydrate, the way it enters your bloodstream may leave you with a sugar high and then a low, whereas a sweet potato, another complex carbohydrate, will leave you with sustained energy. Grapes and bananas, on the other hand, are high in simple sugars, but they're full of important nutrients, and so you're better off choosing them over, say, most "whole wheat" bagels. Here's why: Food manufac-turers understand the complexity of the issue and take advantage of it by mar-keting their products with words like "whole wheat," "whole grain," and "multigrain," leading you to believe that their products are comprised of com-plex carbohydrates. While some of them are, many are not. Look for products that carry a stamp from the Whole Grains Council, and, at the very least, avoid those that have "enriched" in their ingredients list. (When manufacturers have to add something to a product that was there to begin with, food becomes over-processed, taking longer and longer to get from its source to your table.) Also, look for a short ingredients list, always a great sign of a minimally processed food. A true whole grain bagel, bread, or pasta is a good source of complex car-bohydrates and will provide you with sustained energy and insulin levels, avoid-ing those erratic highs and lows associated with eating simple sugars.

3. *Proteins:* Protein is essential for building tissue, but not all proteins are created equal. Seafood is one of the best forms of protein because it has heart-healthy fat

(see Fats, below), but warnings of mercury in fish can get confusing (more on that on page 29). Other great forms of protein are lean poultry and dairy, beef, and eggs, which are all excellent sources of B_{12} vitamins as well (vegans should look at supplementing with a B_{12} vitamin). Eggs have the highest levels of digestibility of all the animal proteins. Dairy products are often recommended for their calcium content, but if you prefer to avoid dairy, you should know that there are plenty of other ways to get your calcium (see Calcium, page 26) and your protein. Beans and other legumes are not only high in protein, but have been found to impact longevity when added to one's diet (so you can be around to see your great-great-grandchildren!). In general, as with other foods, avoid highly processed meats and cheeses, which have more of what you don't want, including additives and bad fats, than what you do want: lean protein.

4. *Fats:* We have learned that there are good fats and bad fats, like our friends the carbohydrates, and you want to be able to distinguish between the two. Omega-3 and omega-6 fatty acids are optimal ingredients for brain development and function. In fact, studies show that omega-3 can impact vision and intelligence, which would explain why baby formulas are enriched with it. Omega-3s are also thought to alleviate postpartum depression. So, you should definitely try to increase your omega-3 intake. Fish remains the highest source of omega-3s, but they are also available in the form of walnuts, flax seed oil, and as supplements. Omega-6 is less talked about because those fatty acids are made from linoleic acid, found in commonly eaten products such as mayonnaise, and in oils such as corn, safflower, sunflower, and cottonseed. In fact, Americans get too much omega-6 in relation to omega-3, and we need to increase our omega-3 intake to balance things out. So while omega-6s are good in theory, you should not look to increase your intake; this is a case of too much of a good thing being bad.

As a general rule of thumb, the less processed your food is, the greater the chance it will contain healthy monounsaturated fats (like olive oil, avocados, and nuts), which are good fats, or polyunsaturated fats (like vegetable oils), which are other good choices. Saturated fats are most often found in animal products and will generally be waxy and solid at room temperature (think of red meat, butter, and whole-milk cheeses). They are best enjoyed in limited quantities, but are not to be avoided.

What I would easily label a "bad," or even "horrible," fat is trans fat. Trans fat will often show up as "partially hydrogenated vegetable oil" in ingredients lists on packaged foods. The process of hydrogenation literally hardens a previously good fat, making it solid at room temperature, so that foods can have a longer shelf life. This is beneficial to food manufacturers and detrimental to the consumer. Your body simply does not know how to deal with this fat. If you can avoid products with hydrogenated vegetable oil and shortening, you will be several steps ahead of the game in terms of the healthy foundation you provide for your baby and yourself.

ABOUT FLAX SEEDS

Flax seeds contain the critical omega-3 fatty acids that are great for the development of baby's brain and vision, for dealing with your postpartum blues, and for your growing children's IQ levels. The omega-3s also help improve your energy level, learning ability, and stress management. Flax seeds must be ground or pressed into oil for you to get all of their benefits, which also include protein and lignan, a type of antioxidant. Ground flax seeds are high in fiber and great in baked goods, such as the Ultimate Bran Muffin (page 202) and Whole Grain Pancakes (page 198). Simply add 1 or 2 tablespoons of ground flax seeds to the dry ingredients. Flax seed oil is great for bolstering shakes such as Vanilla Nut or Creamy Orange Smoothies (see page 208).

5. *Drink a lot of water.* Water, water, water—I cannot say it enough. The recommended amount of water a pregnant woman should drink is six to eight 8-ounce glasses a day, but if you can go eight to ten, do it, especially in the summer. Drinking water will help you with your digestion, reduce constipation, alleviate headaches, decrease swelling, prevent tract infections, and replenish fluid in the amniotic sac. Many of my clients have ended up at the hospital with early onset of contractions brought on by dehydration, so drink up! When you are nursing, drinking water is even more critical for your energy and milk production. Add another two cups to your daily intake, bringing it up to ten to twelve cups a day. The best way to do this is by leaving water bottles all around the house. Every time you see a bottle, drink.

Get Your Daily Nutrients

1. *Folate:* You need 600 micrograms of folate during pregnancy and 500 micrograms while nursing. You can meet that requirement by enjoying foods such as spinach, broccoli, asparagus, peas, beans, avocado, orange juice, bananas, and more. In 1996, the American Food and Drug Administration required the addition of folic acid to enrich breads, cereals, flours, and pastas—the most commonly eaten foods in America. You can get it from those sources, or simply by taking a prenatal vitamin with folic acid in it. But again, I would say that the folate you get from natural sources is preferable to the synthetic version (folic acid).

2. *Calcium:* You need 1,000 milligrams of calcium a day while pregnant and nursing. It is often recommended to get calcium from dairy products, but controversial studies have shown that cow's milk is better absorbed by cows than by people and that the same goes for calcium from dairy products. This is a great example of something that you should research and choose for yourself. If you choose to limit dairy during your pregnancy or while nursing, you should know that there are many opportunities to get calcium from plant-based foods. Kale and broccoli are high in calcium, as are figs, nuts (particularly almonds), and seeds. Beans and tofu are chock-full of calcium, while one tablespoon of powdered nori seaweed will give you 1,200 mg (though I cannot vouch for the taste). Personally, I try to get my calcium from plant-based sources. When I eat cheese, I usually have sheep and goat's milk cheeses because they are easier to digest than cow's milk. But I love cow's milk and cheeses, so I enjoy those on a limited basis.

3. *Iron:* During pregnancy, you need 30 mg of iron daily to produce all the blood needed to bring nutrition to the placenta. Compare this to only 9 mg required during lactation. You will find iron in red meat, poultry, salmon, eggs, tofu, beans, dried fruit, and leafy green vegetables.

Eat Frequently

Eating every two to three hours is helpful for many reasons. If you are suffering from nausea, it will help keep it at bay. Grazing stabilizes your insulin levels, ensuring that you don't go into "starvation" mode, which can trigger uncontrollable cravings. It also increases your metabolism and helps to even out your moods.

Go Organic

Every year our families gather in our home for the Passover Seder, and as they dip into my famous chicken soup, I await their exclamations, "Karen, this is the best chicken soup ever, what makes it taste so good?" I always say that it is my love for them and the positive energy that goes into the preparation, which is true. But this year, my mom came in early to help out. As we prepped for the chicken soup, she said, "You know, I wonder if it is all these organic ingredients that you use that make the soup taste so good." And I think she is right. In fact, most of the food that I prepare at home, and that we prepare at Mothers & Menus, includes fresh, seasonal, organic ingredients, which go a long way in getting me close to a perfect meal, before I even get started cooking.

Let's talk about what *organic* really means: Organic foods are grown without the use of conventional pesticides, artificial fertilizers, or sewage sludge. In the case of animals, it means that they are reared without the use of antibiotics or growth hormones.

Historically, small organic farms were run by people with a deep understanding of the connection between what we eat and how it affects our bodies and our being. However, rapid increases in the demand for organic foods and the nature of supermarket distribution has changed the meaning of *organic* and the standards that define it.

Personally, I do not approach organic as an all-or-nothing choice. In my kitchen you will find a selection of mostly organic foods, with an emphasis on the ones I feel are most critical, such as meat, eggs, dairy, leafy greens, and certain fruits and vegetables, mostly those that won't be peeled or scrubbed before cooking or eating. But I am constantly balancing the ideas of local and organic food. For example, I prefer to buy some nonorganic artisanal cheese from a conscious and committed local farmer, rather than a container of organic cheese that was shipped across the country to the supermarket. That's because I feel this local farmer raised his cows and prepared his cheese with the same positive energy and love with which I infuse my chicken soup—resulting in a product that tastes better and is better for me.

When it comes to meat and eggs, I just feel far more comfortable about organic foodstuff, based on what I have learned. For example, organic eggs are produced by chickens that are allowed to roam free, and eat natural foods, and they do not live in an environment that might promote stress and affect their health.

A gallon of certified organic milk reflects the farm on which it was produced. The dairy cows on that farm were treated humanely, roamed around freely, ate grass, were out in the sun. The cows are not treated with growth hormones or antibiotics. Their milk was acquired in a gentle way, and then, for the most part, pasteurized using a technique that retains some vitamins, minerals, and enzymes that are removed with harsher pasteurization. That is why most regular milk you see is enriched with vitamins and minerals. Remember, when you start with the whole, real food, you do not need to enrich.

Going organic is a personal choice, but see if you can find a way to ease it into your lifestyle, one choice at a time. One way to start is by buying one or more foods from the government's top-twelve list of produce to buy organic, since they are shown to be consistently highest in pesticides and contamination: apples, bell peppers, celery, cherries, grapes (imported), nectarines, peaches, pears, potatoes, raspberries, spinach, and strawberries. At the other end of the spectrum, the following fresh fruits and vegetables consistently have the lowest levels of pesticides: asparagus, avocados, bananas, broccoli, cauliflower, corn (sweet), kiwi, mangos, onions, papayas, pineapples, and peas. Stonyfield Farm has an easy-to-use, wallet-size card with this list, which it keeps updated. You can call 800 PRO-COWS (776-2697), or write to Stonyfield Farm, Wallet Card Offer, 10 Burton Drive, Londonderry, NH 03053. Or visit their Web site at www.stonyfield.com/Organic/EWGShoppersGuide.pdf.

A Word on Foods to Avoid

The list of foods to avoid during pregnancy can be extremely long or very short, depending on your culture, lifestyle, friends and family, where you live, and the doctor you choose. Pregnancy is a great time to define your own "don'ts." Do your research, weigh the pros and cons, and see what resonates with you. Remember that whatever your choice, scientists may find out fifty years from now that a "do" is a "don't" after all, or vice versa, so don't obsess! One great example of that is chicken liver. Fifty years ago advice books for pregnant women strongly recommended eating liver frequently because of its abundance of nutrients along with a mysterious antifatigue factor. Recently, however, women were warned against eating liver while pregnant because it contains vitamin A in excess of the recommended daily intake. Results from studies have been controversial. Jen had cravings for chicken liver with her daughter Jyah (now twenty, smart, strong, and beautiful) and ate it almost daily. Like everything else in your pregnancy, the choice is yours. So make a choice that sits well with you.

Alcohol: As of yet, no one has come up with the definitive amount of alcohol that is safe to drink during pregnancy. Some experts say that a glass a day is okay. Others say pregnant women should avoid it completely since alcohol travels rapidly through the bloodstream and into your placenta, so when you drink, your baby drinks. According to the March of Dimes, alcohol is the most common known cause of damage to developing babies in the United States and is the leading cause of preventable mental retardation. Moderate drinking during pregnancy is still perfectly acceptable in many European countries, but you know that times are changing now that France is putting warning labels on their wine to advise pregnant women about the dangers of alcohol consumption during pregnancy.

Fish High in Mercury: Fish is a notable source of high-quality protein, important nutrients, and the excellent omega-3s. Generally, pregnant women and new moms would do themselves a great service by eating fish two to four times a week. The problem is that fish has mercury in it, which can, in regular doses, harm an unborn child's developing nervous system. Mercury begins with waste dumped in oceans and rivers. Depending on what and where they eat, some fish have much higher traces of mercury than others. Larger fish have been living longer and eat other fish, therefore maintaining a higher accumulation of mercury. Fish can also contain other industrial pollutants, such as polychlorinated biphenyls (PCBs) and bacteria. The U.S. Food and Drug Administration recommends that pregnant women entirely avoid eating shark, swordfish, king mackerel, and tilefish. The March of Dimes adds other fish to that list, including bluefish, tuna steak, striped bass, and freshwater fish. And the Environmental Working Group expands further on the list, limiting canned tuna to once a month. Because the level of mercury in a fish does not depend on the type of fish, but rather on the mercury levels in the area they were caught or raised, check with your local health department to learn about the safest available local choices. You can download a user-friendly, wallet-size list of fish to enjoy (and those to avoid) from oceansalive.org. You may want to update it based on the information that you get from your local fish suppliers.

Highly Processed Foods/Additives: In recent years, food manufacturers have been able to create almost anything in a fat-free, sugar-free, caffeine-free version. But whenever I look at these items, I get extra suspicious—what *is* in it? Normally, a low-fat food will have too much sugar; a sugar-free food will have some sort of chemical replacement; and a low-fat, sugar-free item will be packaged with a list of ingredients too long for me to read (including many words I cannot pronounce). The next time you are drawn to something that seems too good to be true, read the ingredients list. Here is a rule of thumb—the longer the list, the more processed the food is. When in doubt, or in a hurry, pick the product with the fewest ingredients.

Caffeine: I love coffee. Over the course of my journey, I have eliminated many foods from my diet, but I keep going back to my morning cup of Joe. I enjoy it, though, knowing that it is a drug. In fact, coffee is the most widely consumed self-administered drug known to humans (followed by alcohol and nicotine). It is a stimulant that increases your heart rate and can cause nervousness and headaches (as does the withdrawal from it). It also impedes iron absorption and robs the body of calcium (two necessary nutrients during pregnancy) without giving anything in return, as it is an empty-calorie food. Most doctors agree that up to 300 mg of caffeine a day is safe for pregnant women. That includes all forms of caffeine, so check out your own habits: An average cup of brewed coffee contains 150 mg of caffeine, a grande coffee at Starbucks has 400 mg of caffeine, 12 ounces of Diet Coke has 45.6 mg (not to mention sugar substitutes and other harmful additives), 1 ounce of dark chocolate contains 20 mg, and 1 cup of green tea has 15 mg. If you decide to cut coffee out completely, consider going down half a cup a day, week by week, if your withdrawal symptoms—headaches and irritability— are severe. Or, mix decaf with caf, increasing the quantity of decaf until you are down to all decaf. (Look for naturally decaffeinated Swiss Water–processed decaf, as it does not contain the chemicals used to produce other decaf coffees.) If you choose to drink coffee, whether caf or decaf, then make sure to drink 1 cup of water for every cup of coffee to make up for its diuretic properties, which could contribute to dehydration.

My coffee intake varied from pregnancy to pregnancy. I drank one weekly double latte with Nika, half a cup of instant coffee a day with Sophie, and none at all with Ethan because it made me so nauseated. When you are nursing, the caffeine does pass on to your baby through your breast milk, and the same limits of 300 mg are recommended. But you will notice the effects on your baby then: some are directly affected by the caffeine and get cranky and irritable, while others are fine with it. As with everything, check in with your body and your baby to see what works best for you.

Other Foods: Upon becoming pregnant, most women in the Western world are warned by their doctors to avoid a host of additional foods, including unpasteurized or raw-milk cheese; soft or fresh cheese, such as Brie; deli meats and hot dogs; raw or undercooked eggs, fish, and meat; and unpasteurized juices. In general, doctors are trying to prevent exposure to listeria, salmonella, E coli, and other bacteria and pathogens, which can be harmful to the mother but even more harmful to the growing fetus.

Listeria can be found in soil and water and is killed by cooking and pasteurization, hence the recommendation to avoid unpasteurized cheese. However, more outbreaks of listeriosis have been caused by eating contaminated pasteurized cheeses than raw-milk ones; the products in question were made in large-scale industrial factories where contamination occurred after heating but before packaging. Soft cheeses and deli meats provide the right sort of moist environment that listeria loves, which is why they are often listed as foods to avoid unless completely heated through immediately before serving.

Raw or undercooked eggs, fish, and meat can contain salmonella, E coli, and other harmful bacteria that, like listeria, are killed by heat. Ground meat, which is at greater risk for containing bacteria, should always be cooked through completely.

Unpasteurized juices have been linked to some cases of E coli contamination, but then again so have spinach, raspberries, and scallions, all since 2006.

Contrast these dire warnings with customs in other countries: Women in Japan eat sushi; women in France eat raw Camembert. The difference in these cultures is that the sources for their food are fresh: a reputable sushi house or fish monger, and a purveyor of local fresh cheeses. If you look for pristine freshness in your food and food sources, you may need to rely less on the safety net of pasteurization and find yourself trusting foods because of their reputable source.

That said, pregnancy is a time to be conservative. So, for example, if you are uncomfortable in the least with trying out raw cheeses, this would certainly not be a good time to start. While I was very comfortable eating delicious feta cheese salads while pregnant in Greece, at Mothers & Menus, our fresh goat cheeses come from farmers we trust who use pasteurized goat's milk. Alternatively, you can locate a farmer near you who produces artisanal cheese that may not be pasteurized. Nina Planck, author of *Real Food* (Bloomsbury, 2006) and six months pregnant, says, "As long as you trust that your raw cheeses come from a conscientious dairy farmer and a properly inspected or certified or licensed dairy [this varies by state], I think it's perfectly safe to eat raw dairy when you're pregnant. I have eaten raw dairy throughout my pregnancy. Listeria can be found in dairy foods—raw and pasteurized—and in most cases just gives you a bout of food poisoning. The risks of listeriosis to a baby are greater, however, which is why the conventional advice is to avoid young and raw-milk cheeses. For my money, traditional foods, such as raw-milk cheese, in which the good bacteria crowd out the bad, are every bit as safe, if not safer, than the foods of the industrial food chain. This is very much a choice for each pregnant woman to make." I agree. It's all about choices!

Finally, note that once you are nursing, most doctors will lift these restrictions as these foods can no longer potentially jeopardize your baby's health: these bacteria cannot be passed on to your child through breastmilk.

⌘ Real Mothers & Their Menus

The Mothers & Menus service got its name because as I spoke to moms, I realized that every mother needs her own menu. In this chapter you will find stories of real women along with the menus that supported them. See if you hear yourself in their voices and if you can use their menus as guidelines for your own needs. Mostly, though, you can enjoy the honesty with which they share their stories, taking an opportunity to let other mothers know that they are not alone.

Feeling Green

It is estimated that for 90 percent of women who are afflicted by morning sickness, the nausea passes by the twentieth week (and more commonly by week fourteen). For the unlucky 10 percent who experience nausea throughout their entire pregnancy, figuring out what works and what to eat can be very helpful.

With her second pregnancy, Sandra needed a support network around her. That is because during her first pregnancy with daughter Danielle, now six, Sandra was so nauseated, that she was nervous to go through the experience a second time. "Prior to my first pregnancy, I never paid attention to what I was eating from a nutritional standpoint, just in terms of numbers," she explained. "So if I was eating 1,200 calories, I would get 900 of them from a fast-food meal, and the rest in the form of carrots and rice crackers. When I became pregnant with Danielle, I felt like I had gotten a license to eat whatever I craved, which is what I did. I made no correlation between what I was eating and what was going on in my body. I was very nauseous at first, but was reassured by everyone that it would soon pass." As a successful executive at an international PR firm, she found the nausea more than simply uncomfortable. "As a career woman, I was frightened about showing what I think is seen as weakness in the office by employers, colleagues, and clients. Part of the challenge for me was trying to hide the side effects and health effects that I was experiencing: nausea, fatigue, headaches, backaches, ankle aches. So I put my game face on and waited for it to pass."

By the fifth month, Sandra realized that her nausea was not going anywhere, so she started to pay attention to her eating and look for patterns. Although she suffered from morning sickness from morning to night, regardless of what she ate, she soon found that there were certain foods that triggered a more severe reaction—anything fried, greasy, very spicy, and very sweet. In fact, any extremes were the worst culprits. "I realized I had to change my view of eating," Sandra said, "moving beyond satisfying the immediate craving to thinking about how it would affect me afterwards. It was the first time that I had looked at eating from that perspective, and it was a real journey for me. I also realized that I needed to eat often, grazing throughout the day, so I looked for healthy, balanced foods that would work with my nausea, my cravings, and my needs."

Sandra ate rice crackers, soy puffs, and broccoli. She began eating breakfast, which, in an attempt to cut calories, she had never done before. As someone who was already considered overweight prior to her pregnancy, Sandra was scared about gaining more weight, and the doctors reinforced her fears. "They were worried about high blood pressure, increased risk for gestational diabetes, increased risk to the baby, and complications during the delivery," she recounted. "Eventually, I did end up with hypertension, a precursor to preeclampsia, which I wound up developing, which led to a C-section." Although Sandra gained only fifteen pounds throughout most of the pregnancy (and an additional twenty during the last month due to the preeclampsia), she was left traumatized by the experience and was relieved for so many reasons when she finally birthed her beautiful daughter, Danielle.

When Sandra and her husband, Ronen, started talking about a sibling for Danielle, there was more to think about along with the usual considerations. Sandra had left the PR agency to found her own PR firm. Although the firm was growing successfully, it was also cause for concern. "I didn't know how my body would react the second time around," she said, "whether it would be easier, or if possible, worse! Between raising Danielle and growing the company, I shuddered to think about what would happen if I were not able to be around for either of them. It took me five years to prepare myself psychologically."

Shortly after that decision, Sandra got pregnant. The nausea immediately showed up. But this time, she was ready. She shared the news with her employees and asked for their support. She let clients know that she would not be available at all hours, and she enlisted additional help around the home and for Danielle. She started on the antinausea medication early on in her pregnancy and rested more often. Nutritionally, she began using the system that had worked for her with her first pregnancy—grazing throughout the day on healthy, balanced foods. "The pregnancy was considerably easier since I was much more prepared, emotionally, physically, and environmentally with my support system."

Baby Jordan is now four months old. While Sandra was out on maternity leave, her company, Affect Strategies, was recognized by *Working Mother* magazine as one of the twenty-five best small companies for women to work for in the United States. Sandra loves to share her story with other women, so they can learn from her experience. "For me," she offered, "making it through a tough pregnancy is about asking for help and creating a support system—whether it is at work or at home. It is about giving yourself permission to do less and rest more. Whether it is using a food service or asking a friend to help you, ultimately it is about doing whatever you can do to take care of yourself."

	Recommended Menu for Those Suffering from Nausea (follow the Feeling Green variations of the recipes)
Breakfast	Granola Your Way (dry, page 196)
Snack 1	Vanilla Nut Smoothie (page 208)
Lunch	Mushroom Barley Soup (page 62)
Snack 2	Bruschetta with Tapenade (page 102)
Dinner	Seared Chicken Breasts with Balsamic and Herbs (Feeling Green version of Balsamic and Herb–Roasted Chicken, page 120) Roasted Asparagus with Lemon (page 155) Basmati Rice (page 173)

Vegetarian Diet

Vegetarian mothers are often concerned that their diet may not provide enough protein for their babies. In fact, many vegetarians turn to meat during pregnancy because of their own inner cravings. As a vegetarian for over eighteen years, I made no changes to my diet with my first child, introduced fish with my second one, and craved chicken with my third. (Today I am back on a vegetarian diet, though I occasionally eat fish for its health benefits.) Conversely, many carnivore moms find themselves repelled by all forms of meat and chicken and turn to a vegetarian diet, with little information to guide them and some concern about their baby's health.

Doctors agree that a well-rounded vegetarian or vegan diet provides adequate nutrition for the development of a fetus, with an emphasis on *well-rounded*. When following a vegetarian diet, be mindful of nutrients commonly overlooked in a menu free of animal protein, such as protein, B12, and omega-3. You can find these in beans, grains, and fortified products, or look to supplements to increase your intake. One mistake that many vegetarians make (unknowingly) is turning to meat-substitute products to up their protein intake. Many of these products, such as deli "meats," nonchicken nuggets, and ground "beef," contain hydrolyzed soy protein, which almost always contains MSG and sometimes contains genetically modified organisms (GMOs). GMO foods are derived from a relatively new technology, and early research has shown them to be linked to underweight babies and reproductive issues. As with everything, the occasional indulgence of a Tofurkey or similar products within a whole foods–based diet is not harmful and can be extremely satisfying for a carnivore-turned-vegetarian (see the Go Veggie version of Mama's Turkey Meatballs, page 126). Just look for non-GMO or organic soy on the product label (in North America, all produce and products labeled "organic" must be non-GMO).

Recommended Menu for Vegetarians and Vegans	
Breakfast	Whole grain bread with nut butter and sliced apple
Snack 1	Very Berry Smoothie (Feeling Full version for vegans, page 208)
Lunch	Stewed Lentils and Rice (page 136) Mixed greens with Balsamic Vinaigrette (page 73)
Snack 2	Jam Dot Cookie (page 177)
Dinner	Stir-Fried Vegetables with Coconut Curry Sauce (page 137) with Seared Tofu (page 138) over soba noodles

Avoiding Allergens

Given the significant rise in allergies in the United States over the past twenty years, it's no surprise that many pregnant women wonder whether they should avoid allergens, such as peanuts, during pregnancy. In fact, peanuts is the one allergen that the American Academy of Pediatrics recommends that pregnant women avoid regardless of their medical history, because of their allergenic potential. That said, studies show that the rise of clean, antiseptic homes and environments are a huge contributor to a rise in allergies. Since our immune systems don't have any real threats to deal with, they perceive peanuts as a threat. Just something to remember and feel good about when baby starts crawling around on a messy floor that you have not yet gotten around to cleaning!

	Recommended Menu for Women Avoiding Allergens in Their Diet
Breakfast	Quinoa and Amaranth Breakfast Porridge (page 197)
Snack 1	Fresh fruit salad (no strawberries)
Lunch	Roasted Sweet Potato Soup (page 54) White Bean Salad with Olives and Frisée (page 79)
Snack 2	French Lentil Salad (page 78)
Dinner	Grilled Chicken with Summer Salsa (page 118) Basmati and Wild Rice Pilaf (page 165) Green Beans with Carrots, Shallots, and Thyme (page 150)

Fertility Drugs and Weight Gain

For those who have never thought twice about their weight, a weight gain that is off the charts can be quite disconcerting, as was the case for Marie, a pretty, five-foot-nine, thirty-three-year-old investment banker who weighed 135 pounds for most of her life. She is married to her Ivy League football-playing college boyfriend, her partner in work as well as life. The two shared a love of sports and a 5:30 A.M. workout, rain or shine.

Fertility drugs caused several changes in her, both physically and emotionally, including a weight gain of twenty pounds and a beating on her self-esteem. The extra weight, hormones, and complications arising from the fertility process suddenly brought an end to the couple's morning routine. "It was our special time to be alone together," Marie said. "So it was hard for him to see me on several levels—as my husband, as my best friend, and as a workout partner. Suddenly he was so alone."

Marie felt isolated, too. As someone who had spent years taking care of herself through consistent exercise and excellent nutrition, she felt betrayed. As she explained, "Nobody else noticed my weight gain because of my height and build, but I could feel it and I could feel that I was losing my strength. I felt like my body had let me down in so many ways."

After two long years of treatments and complications, Marie and Ted were thrilled to learn that they were pregnant. Marie was cautioned against exercising until a heartbeat was detected in her eighth week, but she was too nauseated to even think about the gym. "Exercise for me was such an endorphin release, and especially with everything going on, I needed it more than ever," she said. By the end of her fourth month, Marie felt good enough to get back to her workout. She took on a trainer and a nutritionist to guide her through the pregnancy, hoping to keep her weight gain under control. "Can you believe it? Even with all of that support, I still gained sixty pounds," she lamented.

Marie was surprised and confused by her body. And while she was happy to go along with whatever was needed in order to grow her long-awaited baby inside of her, the weight gain really affected her in ways beyond the physical.

Similarly, when it came time to take the weight off, Marie was confused by the contradictory feelings of joy in being a new mom, and at the same time a loss of identity. "While I was pregnant, people were very understanding," she said. "But six weeks later, I found myself in a body that I just couldn't recognize." Marie often found herself feeling down and dumpy, sitting on the couch with her Ben & Jerry's. Until then, Ted had been very supportive and understanding, so the change in his attitude caught Marie off guard. "He was so annoyed that I would sit around all day complaining about my weight," she continued, "yet eat ice cream at night. At first I felt so betrayed by him—how could he?" The couple talked it out with a therapist, who helped them recognize each other's point of view. "I finally understood that he wasn't as concerned about my weight gain as he was about the change in my personality. He had married someone confident and sexy, and now I was feeling so insecure and unattractive—it just wasn't connecting to how he saw me," she explained.

Marie weaned Patricia at three months, headed back to work, and got back into her old workout routine. With a lot of support from trainers, Mothers & Menus meals, and her husband, it took Marie ten months to lose fifty-five pounds. She was still fifteen pounds away from her original weight, before she started taking fertility drugs. But Marie's changing body did not deter Marie and Ted from expanding their family. Marie recently gave birth to baby Jack. "Can you believe that pound for pound I gained the exact same amount with Jack as I did with Patricia?" she exclaimed. Marie is waiting to get the green light to exercise again so that she can work on losing those pounds, but she feels differently the second time around. "Now I know how hard it is; I know how my body works," she said. "I am not as surprised as I was before. And also, I have Ted's full support and understanding because we have already made it through this together."

	Recommended Menu for Optimal Eating During Pregnancy*
Breakfast	Ultimate Bran Muffins (page 202)
Snack 1	Whole fruit with nut butter
Lunch	Cup of Creamy Asparagus Soup (page 64) ½ recipe Curried Chicken Salad (page 76) in a wrap
Snack 2	Baked chips with Salsa Cruda (page 96) and Creamy Guacamole (page 98)
Dinner	Broiled Halibut Provençal (page 110) Crisp Roasted Sweet Potatoes (page 169) Spinach, Pine Nuts, and Golden Raisins (page 144)

*If you are carrying twins, add a glass of milk at breakfast or snack time as well as the other half of the Curried Chicken Salad wrap.

Nursing Twins

Once the babies arrive, the menu of a nursing mother of twins has to change dramatically to support Mom, who requires substantially more energy to nourish her babies and function well herself. This was the challenge that Pamela faced very soon after her identical twins were born. "By the time the boys were several days old," she said, "I was so exhausted that when they couldn't latch on, I just gave up." Gave up nursing, that is, but not feeding her children breast milk. Pamela took to the pump.

"It was crazy. I stayed at home for weeks, just pumping, feeding, eating, pumping, and feeding. I felt like I was losing my mind."

To keep up the feeding frenzy, Pamela was told that she needed to eat between 2,800 and 3,000 calories a day. "Three thousand calories just sounded and felt like way too much. I was eating every two hours, and the thought of food was starting to make me queasy," she recalled.

Standing at five feet, ten inches and weighing 118 pounds prepregnancy, Pamela had never thought about when and what to eat. She gained 70 pounds during her pregnancy and was glad that she did. "My boys were born at thirty-six weeks at four pounds fifteen ounces and five pounds five ounces. They did not spend any time in the NICU [neonatal intensive care units] and had no problems. So as much as I struggled with the weight physically and emotionally, it was what my babies and I needed to have a healthy pregnancy."

When the boys were four weeks old, Pamela was forty pounds over her regular weight, eating and pumping continuously, and absolutely drained. Her husband, Mark, urged her to give up the pumping, so that she could catch up on some rest, or be able to leave the house for more than a few minutes at a time. But Pamela was determined. "It just felt like the only thing that I could do for my babies. I kept waiting for that magical bonding moment to happen, and it didn't. Mark had it—but I did not. I felt so guilty. And on top of the guilt, the exhaustion, and the weight, I also had a case of the baby blues."

Pamela and Mark, both researchers, had read and studied just about every book on pregnancy after learning that they were expecting. "But nothing had prepared me for this," Pamela said. "I don't think anyone really talks about the range of emotions that you can feel after you have the baby. Or maybe they do and I just skipped over that part. I am not sure. I am just so lucky that I had Mark's support throughout. He was able to hold my space while I went through my ups and downs."

When the boys were twelve weeks old, Pamela weaned them onto formula and began to leave the house, alone. "I realized that I just needed some time to myself. I don't need much, but when I have that, I can really be present when I am with them. But I have to say that even when they are not around, I worry and think about them all the time." Physically, Pamela is back to her prepregnancy weight, but not without effort. "I am at the gym five days a week and people tell me I look great, but I find it strange that I actually have to think about what I am eating. Before, I could just walk into a restaurant and order the steak and french fries. Now I have to look at the menu for healthier alternatives. I guess it is all part of the learning." Most of all, Pamela is still amazed at how much their lives have changed. "I can't believe I am a mother to twins. Identical twins! It is really incredible. They are starting to discover and relate to each other now. It is just astonishing to watch them."

	Recommended Menu for a Mother Nursing Twins
Breakfast	Whole Grain Pancakes (page 198) with Balsamic-Macerated Strawberries (page 187)
Snack 1	Chocolate–peanut butter smoothie (Feeling Food version, page 209)
Lunch	Miso Soup over soba noodles (Feeling Food version, page 59) Crab Salad with Cilantro and Chives (page 75) on whole grain bread
Snack 2	Fresh fruit with cheese
Dinner	Seared Beef Tenderloin with Port and Mushrooms (page 122) Potato and Celery Root Puree (page 171) Sautéed Kale (page 147)
Snack 3	Ultra-Energy Bar (page 180)

Of course, if you have "just" one baby to nurse, you would follow a similar menu but cut out one of the snacks or just eat smaller portions of everything on the menu. While you are nursing, you often feel ravenous, as if you could just keep eating and eating. When filling up on these nutritious, fiber-rich whole foods, you will be able to fill the bottom of that pit and know that you are providing yourself with sustained energy. Whatever you do, do not ignore your hunger. This is a sure sign from your body that it needs something—more nutrients, larger portions, or sometimes, sleep.

Weight Loss

"Take care of yourself, take care of yourself, take care of yourself" is Charli Bohm's mantra. Mother to Sara, fourteen, Max, ten, and Jacob, two, Charli knows all about the importance of attending to yourself so that you can care for others in your life. While she was pregnant with Jacob, she set about putting structures in place, ordering a laundry service, arranging meals from Mothers & Menus, and asking her housekeeper to help out for an additional day a week. By the time Jacob came along, Charli was ready for almost anything and up for the challenging time ahead of losing all the weight she had gained in her pregnancy. "When we started telling people we were pregnant, my ex-husband called me up and said, 'Did you tell Eric how big you get?' It was funny because it was so true! Although I gained only twenty-five pounds with Sara and snapped right back to my size two, with Max I had gained seventy pounds. I was prepared for it to go that way again because I was pregnant with a boy and older than when I had Sara." She did prepare her husband, Eric, who was fully nurturing and supportive as he watched her transformation. This time, Charli wanted to be ready, so unlike during her pregnancy with Max, she ate well and exercised—and gained the same seventy pounds. "I just knew that this is what my body needs and what my baby needs, so I had no problems with it at all," she said.

When it came time to losing the weight, Charli already had an idea of what it would take. "With Max, I had lost some weight early on, but kept on an additional forty-five pounds, which did not come off until after I stopped nursing." For Charli that meant at least nine months, the length of time she had committed to breast-feeding her child. "The first time around I was really upset," she said. "And people's comments did not do much to help. The rule of thumb is that you will lose your weight while breastfeeding. Well, apparently, that doesn't work for everyone. The hormone adjustment is so individual—some people might lose the weight right away, but others, like me, might hold onto it, for whatever reason their body needs it. With your first baby, if you are not following the charts for gaining weight and losing it, and your baby is crying, and you are nursing all the time, and you are exhausted, you can start to freak out and think—this is it?"

With Jacob, Charli knew her body's routine, so she started working out after the six-week checkup and continued to eat well postpartum. She expected to be rewarded for all of her efforts, and showed up at her annual checkup expectantly. She got on the scale only to find that she weighed exactly the same as she had at her six-week checkup. Charli was frustrated. "I knew I could lose it and this is just my body's way of being. The difference was that this time I was eight years older. There is a big difference between thirty and thirty-eight. It was a lot harder. I did start to get nervous that maybe this time I would not get my body back."

Charli persevered with her conscientious eating and exercise and within four months was back into her old jeans. "It is almost as if my body has some trigger from the hormones. It keeps thinking I am pregnant and just keeps the weight on," she said. "I am just so happy to be myself again." But even after dropping the weight, Charli felt herself go into a fog. Between caring for her family, struggling with her weight loss, and going back to work, Charli had gotten lost. "I realized that somewhere along the way, I lost sight of my own mantra. I was so busy taking care of Jacob and making sure that everyone else was taken care of, that somewhere in there I forgot to take care of me." Together with Eric, she created a schedule that would give Charli some time to herself. "You have to find the balance between what makes you happy as a woman, and what you want to give your child, because that is what gives you the strength to be the best parent you can be," she declared.

	Recommended Menu for Getting Back to Your Prepregnancy Weight
Breakfast	Tomato, Herb, and Goat Cheese Frittata (page 194)
Snack 1	Mixed nuts
Lunch	Carrot Soup with Coriander, Curry, Ginger, and Chives (page 48) Baby Spinach Salad with Pears, Toasted Walnuts, and Pecorino (page 74)
Snack 2	White Bean Dip with Crudités (page 95)
Dinner	Miso-Glazed Salmon (page 114) Sautéed Bitter Greens with Shallots (page 152) Quinoa with Mushrooms, Caramelized Squash, and Toasted Pecans (page 164)

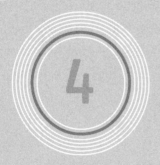

Soups

We serve soup every day to our Mothers & Menus clients because soups are warm, nurturing, and easy to absorb. They are an especially good choice for expectant women in their first or last trimester who are feeling green or full, for moms recovering from cesarean sections with difficulties digesting as a result, and for nursing moms of fussy babies. Also, if you are not up to eating raw vegetables, you can get your vitamins and minerals via your soup.

In Chinese medicine, warm foods are recommended because of their effect on the spleen, which transforms food into energy. Adding a warm soup to your salad or sandwich at lunch or dinner may give you more energy and ease your digestion, making life easier for you and your baby. If your growing baby seems more uncomfortable and active at night, try this out: enjoy a fuller breakfast, lunch, and snacks, and have one of these hearty soups for a dinner that will tide you over until the morning without leaving you feeling too full.

If you don't have a hand blender in your kitchen, I strongly recommend investing in one (about $35 at any housewares or kitchen supply store for a basic model). Also called an immersion blender, this tool lets you blend hot soups and sauces right in the pot, which is not only fast but also means you'll have fewer dishes to do because you're not washing a ladle, a blender, and a second pot to put the pureed soup into. You'll also get plenty of use out of it when baby comes and you need to puree small batches of food.

Finally, keep in mind that these soups can be made in advance, and refrigerated or even frozen (see page 65), and then reheated so they are ready when you are.

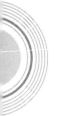

Carrot Soup with Coriander, Curry, Ginger, and Chives • MAKES ABOUT 2 QUARTS OR 4 SERVINGS

This beautiful, delicious, bright orange soup is a huge favorite with our customers. The exotic blend of spices adds depth to the familiar carrot, complementing and enhancing its natural sweet flavor. Enjoy leftovers hot or cold, which is a great option for when you have just a few minutes to sip something nutritious.

2 tablespoons olive oil

1 medium sweet onion, chopped

1 medium Yukon Gold potato, peeled and chopped

1 clove garlic, chopped

1 tablespoon peeled and grated fresh ginger

1 teaspoon ground coriander

1 teaspoon curry powder

1½ pounds carrots, peeled and chopped

4 cups chicken or vegetable stock, homemade (page 66 or 67)
   or store-bought, or water

Salt and freshly ground pepper

½ cup heavy cream, optional

½ cup chopped fresh chives, optional

Heat the olive oil in a large saucepan over medium heat. Add the onion, potato, garlic, ginger, coriander, and curry powder and cook until the onion is soft and translucent, 5 to 8 minutes. Add the carrots and stock and bring to a boil. Reduce the heat, cover, and simmer for 20 minutes, or until the carrots are tender.

Puree in a blender and season to taste with salt and pepper. Swirl in the cream, if desired, and garnish with the chives, if using, before serving.

FEELING GREEN: The fresh gingerroot in this soup may prove to be quite helpful. Increase the ginger by 1 teaspoon and omit the chives. Try taking small sips of the soup (at room temperature) throughout the day.

FEELING FOOD: Definitely go for the cream option and enjoy—this sweet and creamy soup is a fabulous, comforting treat.

FEELING FULL: Omit the potato and prepare the soup as directed. Substitute plain, low-fat yogurt, if desired, for the cream.

BABY FOOD

Once you have successfully introduced your baby to solids and are looking to expand his repertoire, consider pureeing the following soups for him:

- Carrot Soup with Coriander, Curry, Ginger, and Chives
- Sweet Pea and Mint Soup
- Roasted Sweet Potato Soup
- Grounding Soup
- Mushroom Barley Soup
- Creamy Asparagus Soup

Hold back on the salt and pepper when making these, but not the herbs; those are fine. Reserve some soup for him (puree if the soup is not already smooth), and then season the rest to taste for you and the family. With the exception of Mushroom Barley and Creamy Asparagus soups, which do not freeze well, freeze the pureed soups in ice cube trays. Drop one or two cubes into a resealable sandwich bag. Defrost for an easy, nutritious baby meal on the go.

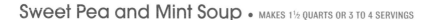

Sweet Pea and Mint Soup • MAKES 1½ QUARTS OR 3 TO 4 SERVINGS

With its beautiful bright green color and sweet pea flavor, this soup is as pretty and delicious as it is good for you. If you do not plan to serve it immediately, cool the base for 30 minutes before adding the peas and herbs. This will allow you to preserve the soup's gorgeous hue. When reheating, cook for 5 minutes and then puree before serving.

1 tablespoon olive oil

1 small sweet onion, chopped

1 medium Yukon Gold potato, peeled and cut into ½-inch chunks

1 medium leek, white and green parts, chopped, optional

4 cups vegetable stock, homemade (page 67) or store-bought, or water

1 (10-ounce) package frozen peas

½ cup fresh mint leaves, or 2 tablespoons fresh dill

Salt and freshly ground pepper

Heat the olive oil in a large saucepan over medium heat. Add the onion, potato, and leek, if using, and cook, stirring occasionally, until the onion is soft and translucent, 5 to 8 minutes.

Add the vegetable stock and bring to a boil. Reduce the heat and simmer, covered, until the potato is tender, about 20 minutes.

Add the peas and return to a simmer. Cook for 5 minutes, or until the peas are tender. Add the mint and puree in a blender. Season with salt and pepper to taste.

FEELING GREEN: This one is a little tricky. If you are feeling just a little green, then this soup with its mild flavors and the nausea-relieving properties of fresh mint may be soothing. Just omit the onion and optional leek and prepare as directed, but make sure to use vegetable stock, not water, or you will be left with terrifically bland food for your baby, but nothing quite pleasing enough for your own palate. However, if you are fully green, then I would recommend a different soup because peas may cause bloating, which can make you even greener. Try the Feeling Green variations of the Roasted Sweet Potato Soup (page 54) or Mushroom Barley Soup (page 62).

FEELING FOOD: Add a handful of whole grain croutons for a smooth and crunchy contrast.

FEELING FULL: Prepare the soup as directed, but omit the potato. The soup will still retain its rich consistency.

ABOUT LEEKS

A leek has more than twice the amount of iron as a cup of green vegetables. So even though it is optional in the recipe, try to include it. But remember that the leek is a member of the onion family, so if you are not doing well with onions or if your breastfed baby is a little fussy, go without for now.

Curried Butternut Squash Soup • MAKES 2 QUARTS OR 4 SERVINGS

This tasty, warming soup is filled with nutrients from the vegetables and also from the curry powder, which is actually a mix of powders that generally includes turmeric, coriander, chiles, cumin, pepper, ginger, cinnamon, cassia, and clove. Turmeric is the most potent of the mix, with antioxidants and antiseptics, which strengthen the stomach and help with digestion.

2 tablespoons olive oil

1 medium sweet onion, chopped

1 large carrot, chopped

1 stalk celery, chopped

1 large shallot, sliced

1 medium butternut squash, peeled, seeded, and cut into 1-inch chunks

2 tablespoons curry powder

1 bay leaf

6 cups vegetable stock, homemade (page 67) or store-bought, or water

Salt and freshly ground pepper

Chopped scallions, white and green parts for garnish

Fresh cilantro leaves for garnish

Heat the olive oil in a large saucepan over medium heat. Add the onion, carrot, celery, and shallot and cook until the onion is translucent and soft, 5 to 8 minutes.

Add the squash and curry powder to the pan and cook for 5 more minutes, stirring well to coat the vegetables with the curry. Add the bay leaf and stock and bring to a boil. Lower the heat and simmer, covered, for 30 minutes, or until the squash is very tender.

Discard the bay leaf and puree the soup in a blender. Season to taste with salt and pepper. Garnish with chopped scallions and cilantro before serving.

FEELING GREEN: Omit the onion and scallions and replace the curry powder with 2 teaspoons ground cinnamon and 1 teaspoon turmeric.

FEELING FOOD: Panfry 1 slice of turkey bacon per serving until crisp, and chop and add to the soup for a heartier, enriched bowlful.

FEELING FULL: Reduce the oil to 1 tablespoon and continue to follow the recipe as is. This creamy soup is deceptively rich, given its clean, nutritious ingredients.

 LEGEND HAS IT . . .

In India, turmeric has been an active ingredient in cosmetics for centuries because of its healing effects on dry or discolored skin. Even today, one Indian parenting Web site advises women to do the following prior to conception: Apply a mixture of turmeric and *malai* (clotted cream) to your stomach before bathing. Leave on for 15 minutes and wash off with soap. Reapply after bathing, and leave on for 5 minutes, washing off only with water. Wipe your stomach gently with a towel when drying it. According to the Web site, the sooner you start this routine, the more supple and elastic your skin will become, and after giving birth, you will not be left with stretch marks.

Roasted Sweet Potato Soup • MAKES 2 QUARTS OR 4 TO 6 SERVINGS

Because this soup is naturally sweet and rich, many of our clients enjoy it at the end of their dinner to stave off dessert cravings. Roasting the potatoes requires a couple of extra steps—and therefore extra time—but it really enhances the taste of the soup (for a shortcut, check out Express, opposite). Another reason to roast rather than boil them is that the nutrients of sweet potatoes are found close to their skin. Baking them in their skins ensures the maximum intake of the nutrients they offer, including vitamins A, C, and E.

6 plum tomatoes, halved and seeded
4 garlic cloves, minced
¼ cup olive oil
3 large sweet potatoes, skin on, halved
1 medium sweet onion, chopped
1 medium carrot, chopped
1 stalk celery, chopped
2 quarts vegetable stock, homemade (page 67) or store-bought, or water
1 tablespoon chopped fresh thyme
2 tablespoons chopped fresh chives
Salt and freshly ground pepper
Chopped fresh Italian parsley for garnish

Preheat the oven to 425°F.

Toss the tomatoes with half of the garlic and 1 tablespoon of the olive oil in a baking dish. Roast for 30 minutes, or until they are soft and slightly shriveled. Set aside to cool.

While the tomatoes are baking, put the sweet potatoes, cut side down, in a large baking dish and drizzle with 1 tablespoon of the olive oil. Bake until the potatoes are tender, 20 to 25 minutes. Set aside to cool.

Heat the remaining 2 tablespoons of olive oil in a large saucepan over medium heat. Add the onion, carrot, celery, and remaining garlic and cook until the onion is translucent and begins to caramelize, about 8 minutes.

Remove the skins from the sweet potatoes and add the flesh to the pot along with the stock. Bring to a boil, lower the heat, and simmer for 30 minutes.

Meanwhile, chop the tomatoes into small pieces and set aside.

Add the thyme and chives to the soup and puree in a blender until smooth. Season with salt and pepper and garnish with tomatoes and chopped parsley before serving.

Express: When you are short on time, use this version for a faster yet still nutritious and delicious soup: Omit the tomatoes and peel the sweet potatoes and cut into 1-inch chunks. Skip the roasting step and sauté the sweet potatoes along with the onion, carrot, and celery. Proceed with the rest of the recipe as directed.

FEELING GREEN: Omit the garlic and tomatoes. The gentle, smooth texture of this soup should be soothing.

FEELING FOOD: Toast 2 tablespoons of pine nuts (see page 70) and add to the soup after blending.

FEELING FULL: Enhance this soup's nutrient level further by adding a handful of chopped kale or fresh spinach in the last 5 to 10 minutes of cooking.

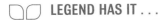 **LEGEND HAS IT . . .**

In Hawaii, where sweet potatoes are called *uala*, expectant women are given tonic from their leaves for a healthful pregnancy, and nursing mothers eat them to induce lactation.

Italian Lentil Soup • MAKES 2 QUARTS OR 4 TO 6 SERVINGS

This thick and hearty soup is quick, easy, and tremendously satisfying. Lentils are an excellent source of protein, folate, and fiber, and because they are small, they are easier to digest than other legumes. This soup improves with age, just like us. Sitting overnight in the refrigerator will actually bring out its flavor. At eighteen months, my son Ethan loves this soup with some brown rice.

  2 tablespoons olive oil
  1 medium sweet onion, diced
  2 medium carrots, peeled and diced
  1 stalk celery, diced
  2 cloves garlic, minced
  1 bay leaf
  2 sprigs fresh thyme
  2 cups green or brown lentils, rinsed
  1 (16-ounce) can plum tomatoes, crushed, with their juices
    Salt and freshly ground pepper

Heat the olive oil in a large saucepan over medium heat. Add the onion, carrots, celery, and garlic and cook until the onion is translucent, 5 to 8 minutes. Add the bay leaf, thyme, and lentils and cook for 1 minute. Add the tomatoes and 6 cups of cold water and bring to a boil. Reduce the heat, cover, and simmer for about 40 minutes, or until the lentils are tender.

Discard the bay leaf and thyme. Season to taste with salt and pepper.

In a pinch: If you do not have any lentils around, this soup works beautifully with split peas. Simply replace the lentils with split peas and prepare exactly as directed.

FEELING GREEN: Omit the onions, garlic, and tomatoes, and add 1 tablespoon of ground ginger. Prepare as directed, pureeing the soup for greater digestibility.

FEELING FOOD: Pour a ladleful of this soup over ½ cup of cooked brown or basmati rice for a heartier meal.

FEELING FULL: Skip the oil and the sautéing. Combine all of the ingredients together in the saucepan and proceed with the simmering as directed. Now you have a high-protein, high-fiber, completely fat-free soup.

Grounding Soup •

This soothing soup has a notably calming effect and is perfect for anyone (male or female) feeling anxious or nervous. It is also helpful when nursing, as it promotes lactation and balances blood sugar. Another benefit? The combination of all these vegetables is simply delicious.

2 tablespoons olive oil

1 medium sweet onion, chopped

1 medium leek, white part only, chopped

1 clove garlic, chopped

1 stalk celery, chopped

1 medium carrot, peeled and chopped

1 medium Yukon Gold potato, peeled and chopped

1 medium sweet potato, peeled and chopped

1 medium parsnip, peeled and chopped

1 medium turnip or small rutabaga, peeled and chopped

1 small pumpkin or butternut or kabocha squash, peeled and chopped

1 bay leaf

2 quarts chicken or vegetable stock, homemade (page 66 or 67) or store-bought, or water

1 tablespoon finely chopped fresh thyme, or ½ teaspoon dried thyme

Salt and freshly ground pepper

In a large saucepan, heat the oil over medium heat. Add the onion, leek, garlic, celery, and carrot and cook until the onion is translucent, 5 to 8 minutes. Add both potatoes, the parsnip, turnip, pumpkin, and bay leaf. Stir and then pour in the stock. Bring to a boil, reduce the heat, and simmer, uncovered, until the vegetables are tender, about 20 minutes.

Add the thyme and puree the soup in a blender. Season with salt and pepper to taste.

FEELING GREEN: Prepare without the onion and leek, choose stock over water, and enjoy this calming soup, which will also help out with digestion.

FEELING FOOD: While the soup is simmering, peel and cube 1 beet and sauté in olive oil over medium heat until tender and slightly crispy, 8 to 10 minutes. Drain well on paper towels and add to the soup for a satisfying crunch.

FEELING FULL: Replace the Yukon Gold potato with a sweet potato, or omit the potatoes entirely.

Miso Soup • MAKES 1 QUART OR 2 TO 3 SERVINGS

There are just two foods that I will gently push a new mom to try out while she is nursing, and miso soup is one of them (the other is kale, page 147). That is because it is so helpful for digestion for both mom and baby (see About Miso, opposite). See if you can work a cup of miso soup into your diet once or twice a week. This recipe will make it worthwhile. When choosing your paste, look for light or red miso for most of the year, and go darker and heartier for the cold winter months. You can find dried wakame seaweed in convenient packages (Eden sells them in 2.1-ounce packages) in the Asian section of some supermarkets, at health food stores, and at any Asian specialty store.

4 cups vegetable stock, homemade (page 67) or store-bought, or water
1 (6-inch) piece dried wakame seaweed
1 small carrot, peeled and cut into matchsticks
½ cup thinly sliced bok choy or napa or green cabbage
½ cup diced firm tofu
2 to 3 tablespoons red or light miso paste, to taste
2 tablespoons finely chopped scallions, white and green parts, optional

Bring the stock to a boil in a medium saucepan. Remove from the heat and add the wakame to the pan. Let soak until softened, about 20 minutes.

Remove the wakame with a slotted spoon, cut into bite-size pieces, and return to the pan. Return the stock to a boil and then lower the heat and simmer for 10 minutes. Add the carrot and bok choy and cook for 1 minute. Add the tofu.

Remove a cup of the stock and add the miso paste to it. Stir to dissolve the miso and then stir the mixture back into the pan. Heat the soup over medium heat until small bubbles begin to form around the edge of the pan. Do not boil. Garnish with scallions before serving.

FEELING GREEN: Pour 1 cup of very hot water over 1 tablespoon of miso paste in a mug. Stir in some diced tofu if you feel up to it.

FEELING FOOD: Pour 1 cup of soup over a cup of cooked soba noodles for a delicious, super-nutritious noodle treat.

FEELING FULL: Don't change a thing. This nutrient-dense, low-calorie soup is a great, satisfying addition to your daily diet.

ABOUT MISO

Miso paste is a smooth, dark puree made from soybeans, fermented barley or rice, and sea salt, which have aged together over a period of several months to several years. It provides a nutritious balance of complex carbohydrates, essential oils, protein, vitamins, and minerals. Miso contains living enzymes that help digest food, lower cholesterol, and increase friendly bacteria (especially helpful when taking antibiotics). To keep these enzymes alive, miso is never boiled during cooking. According to Japanese legend, miso was a gift from the gods to ensure humanity's health, longevity, and happiness.

Cold and Flu Season Soup · MAKES 2 QUARTS OR 4 TO 6 SERVINGS

Being sick is bad enough under any circumstance, but when you are pregnant or nursing and trying to avoid medication, you need a helping hand to get back on your feet. This soup is just what the doctor ordered. Cayenne pepper stimulates circulation, aids in digestion, and breaks up congestion, making it the perfect over-the-stove remedy for your cold. So rest up, enjoy, and feel better! Often water substitutes well for stock, but in this case, the properties of the chicken soup are essential for your recovery.

1½ quarts chicken stock, homemade (page 66) or store-bought
1 tablespoon peeled and grated fresh ginger
1 tablespoon minced garlic
½ teaspoon cayenne pepper
2 cups thinly sliced kale leaves
2 cups diced cooked chicken
1 tablespoon finely chopped scallion, white and green parts

Combine the stock, ginger, garlic, and cayenne in a large saucepan over low heat. Bring to a simmer and cook for 15 minutes.

Increase the heat to medium, add the kale, and cook for 5 minutes. Add the chicken and cook for 1 or 2 minutes to heat through.

Top with scallions before serving.

FEELING GREEN: Add another teaspoon of ginger to the stock and omit the cayenne, kale, and scallions. (Chicken is optional, depending on how you are feeling about it today.) Cayenne is great for curing the common cold, but can aggravate your nausea, so leave it out.

FEELING FOOD: Ladle this soup over a bowl of cooked egg noodles.

FEELING FULL: Among its many benefits, cayenne pepper is also known for raising metabolism, so enjoy!

Creamy Tomato Basil Soup • MAKES 2 QUARTS OR 4 TO 6 SERVINGS

This velvety soup does not have an ounce of cream, achieving its "faux" creamy texture from the potato. This comforting, nourishing soup may remind you of a childhood favorite, but the added fiber, vitamins, and minerals are very adult, and the two-step recipe makes it almost as fast as pouring some out of a can.

2 tablespoons olive oil

1 medium sweet onion, cut into 1-inch chunks

1 large carrot, chopped

1 small Yukon Gold potato, chopped

1 medium shallot, chopped

1 bay leaf

1 (28-ounce) can whole plum tomatoes, with their juice

2 cups vegetable stock, homemade (page 67) or store-bought, or water

½ cup fresh basil leaves, chopped

Salt and freshly ground pepper

In a large pot, heat the olive oil over medium heat. Add the onion, carrot, potato, and shallot and cook until the onion is translucent, 5 to 8 minutes. Add the bay leaf, tomatoes, and stock and bring to a boil. Reduce the heat, cover, and simmer until the carrots and potatoes are tender, about 30 minutes.

Discard the bay leaf. Puree the soup in a blender until smooth. Stir in the basil and season with salt and pepper.

FEELING GREEN: When adding the tomatoes and stock, add 1 tablespoon of honey to balance the acidity of the tomatoes.

FEELING FOOD: Sprinkle grated cheese over Crostini (page 102) or spread with goat cheese, and broil in the oven until melted. Then add to the soup.

FEELING FULL: Reduce the oil to 1 tablespoon and omit the potato. After pureeing the soup, add chopped spinach and heat through on medium heat until just wilted.

Mushroom Barley Soup • MAKES ABOUT 2 QUARTS OR 4 TO 6 SERVINGS

This wonderful fall and winter soup is unbelievably rich in nutrients. The immunity-building mushrooms are high in vitamins, minerals, and folic acid, and barley is packed with dietary fiber, selenium, and antioxidants. Above all, this soup tastes great.

1/4 ounce dried mushrooms, such as porcini, shiitake, or black trumpet
3 tablespoons olive oil
1 pound cremini mushrooms, sliced
8 ounces shiitake mushrooms, trimmed and sliced
2 small shallots, chopped
1 small leek, white and green parts, chopped
1 small sweet onion, chopped
1 stalk celery, diced
1 medium carrot, diced
1/2 cup pearled barley
4 cups chicken or vegetable stock, homemade (page 66 or 67) or store-bought
1 sprig fresh thyme
1 bay leaf
1 tablespoon chopped fresh dill
Salt and freshly ground pepper

Put the dried mushrooms in a bowl. Bring 1 cup of water to a boil and pour over the mushrooms. Let soak for 20 to 30 minutes.

Drain the dried mushrooms, reserving their liquid. Chop the mushrooms.

In a large saucepan, heat the oil over medium heat. Add the chopped dried mushrooms to the pot along with the cremini and shiitake mushrooms, shallots, leek, onion, celery, carrot, and barley. Increase the heat to medium-high and cook the vegetables, stirring often, until the mushrooms have browned and the vegetables are beginning to soften, about 10 minutes.

Strain the soaking liquid from the mushrooms and add it to the pot along with the stock, thyme, and bay leaf. Bring to a boil, reduce the heat, and simmer until the barley is tender, about 40 minutes.

If the soup is too thick, add water to thin it to the desired consistency. Remove the thyme and bay leaf, sprinkle with dill, and season with salt and pepper to taste. Serve immediately.

FEELING GREEN: Barley-based foods are thought to ease nausea, so try this soup as is, but if the dried or shiitake mushrooms sound too exotic right now, replace them with additional creminis or white button mushrooms.

FEELING FOOD: Prepare creamy mushroom soup instead: Omit the barley. Decrease the stock to 3 cups, and add an optional ¼ cup of dry sherry. Decrease the simmering time to 30 minutes. Remove the thyme and bay leaf, and puree in a blender, leaving the soup with a little texture.

FEELING FULL: Use the Feeling Food variation to skip the barley and enjoy a lighter, creamier treat.

LEGEND HAS IT . . .

A three thousand—year-old Egyptian document holds one of the earliest written records of a pregnancy test. The papyrus described a test in which a woman who might be pregnant would plant wheat and barley seeds instead of a stick. What determined the "blue line"? If the barley grew, it meant she was pregnant with a boy; if the wheat grew, she would bear a girl. And if neither grew, she was not pregnant. A test of this theory in 1963 found the pregnancy aspect to be accurate 70 percent of the time (but not the gender determination). In ancient China, barley was honored as a symbol of male virility since the heads of barley are heavy and contain numerous seeds.

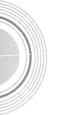

Creamy Asparagus Soup • MAKES 2½ QUARTS OR 6 SERVINGS

This soup is a staple in our house in spring and summer. Its mild but intriguing flavors make it appeal-ing to kids as well as adults. Select asparagus with a bright green hue and closed, compact tips. Although the pencil-thin variety get all of the attention, you can opt for stalks with a large diameter here since they will be pureed.

Remember that leeks are a member of the onion family, so if you or your nursing baby is sensitive to onions right now, omit them (see the Feeling Green variation, opposite).

¼ cup olive oil
1 medium sweet onion, chopped
1 stalk celery, chopped
2 leeks, white and green parts, chopped
3 medium Yukon Gold potatoes, peeled and chopped
2 bay leaves
2 quarts chicken or vegetable stock, homemade (page 66 or 67),
    or store-bought
2 pounds medium asparagus (approximately 2 bunches)
    Salt and freshly ground pepper

In a large saucepan, heat the oil over medium heat. Add the onion, celery, leeks, and potatoes and cook, stirring frequently, until the vegetables are tender, about 10 minutes. Add the bay leaves.

Meanwhile, in a medium saucepan, bring the stock to a boil over high heat. Break off the tough ends from the asparagus and discard. Cut the asparagus stalks into 1-inch pieces and add to the stock. Boil for 1 minute until slightly tender but still bright green. Remove the asparagus from the stock with a slotted spoon (you will be using the stock in a moment, so keep it hot) and transfer them to a colander. Run cold water over them to stop the cooking. Set aside.

Pour the boiling stock over the leek and potato mixture and simmer, lowering the heat if necessary, until the potatoes are tender, about 20 minutes. Remove the bay leaves.

Reserve 1 cup of the asparagus tips for garnish and add the remaining pieces to the soup. Puree in a blender until smooth. Season with salt and pepper and serve immediately, garnished with the reserved asparagus tips.

FEELING GREEN: Reduce the oil to 2 tablespoons and omit the onion and the leek. Top the soup with plain croutons for some crunch.

FEELING FOOD: Bring this soup back to its traditional roots: replace the olive oil with butter, choose chicken stock over vegetable, and add 2 tablespoons of heavy cream per serving.

FEELING FULL: Reduce the oil to 2 tablespoons and omit the potatoes. You will end up with a thinner consistency, which you may want to fill out by stirring in some low-fat plain yogurt.

ABOUT ASPARAGUS

If you are trying to get pregnant or are in your early stages of pregnancy, then this is the soup for you. One cup of asparagus has more folate (naturally occurring folic acid) than 4 cups of raw spinach.

FREEZING SOUP

My dad, Joe, insists that soups taste better after being frozen. I don't always agree, but I can't argue against the ease of pulling something out of the freezer for a quick, nourishing lunch or dinner. The following soups freeze well. Consider making double batches and freezing them in 32-ounce containers (serves 2) so that you are never far away from a hot (and according to my dad, tastier) meal:

Carrot Soup with Coriander, Curry, Ginger, and Chives

Roasted Sweet Potato Soup

Italian Lentil Soup

Grounding Soup

Cold and Flu Season Soup

Creamy Tomato Basil Soup

If possible, defrost gently in your fridge overnight before reheating in a saucepan over low heat until simmering. Note that a soup's consistency may change when it is frozen and reheated. Vegetable-based soups will be more watery, whereas bean-based soups will thicken (add a little water if needed). All of these soups will still taste great, though.

Chicken Stock • MAKES 3 QUARTS

This chicken stock takes less than 1 hour to prepare (including cooking time) and leaves you with one whole poached chicken, perfect for chicken salad (page 76) or soup (page 60). In fact, this is the recipe I turn to as the base of my homemade chicken soup. I gently simmer diced vegetables—celery, carrots, and potato, of course, but also sweet potato and butternut squash—in the stock before returning the cooked chicken to the pot and showering everything with handfuls of chopped parsley.

1 tablespoon olive oil

1 medium yellow onion, quartered

1 medium carrot, cut into 2 chunks

1 stalk celery, cut into 2 chunks

1 clove garlic, left whole

1 bay leaf

2 sprigs fresh thyme

2 stems fresh Italian parsley, with leaves

8 whole black peppercorns

1 (3½-pound) chicken

Heat the olive oil in a large saucepan over medium heat. Add the onion, carrot, celery, and garlic and cook until the onion is translucent, 5 to 8 minutes. Add the bay leaf, thyme, parsley, peppercorns, chicken, and 3 quarts (12 cups) of cold water. Bring almost to a boil and then reduce the heat. Simmer, uncovered, until the chicken is cooked through, about 40 minutes. Skim the surface often with a ladle while the stock is cooking to remove fat and anything that would cloud the liquid, to ensure a clear stock.

Remove the chicken and set aside to cool. Remove the meat from the bones and skin and reserve for other uses. Discard the skin and bones.

Strain the stock into containers. Let cool completely, then cover and refrigerate for up to 5 days or freeze for up to 1 month. Refrigerate overnight and skim off any fat before freezing.

Vegetable Stock • MAKES 2 QUARTS

While I used to think of stock as yet another step in soup preparation, I now see it as a great opportunity to use up all of those vegetables lurking in the refrigerator. Homemade stock enhances the flavor of your recipes, increases their nutritional value, and alleviates guilt! Consider adding a handful of fresh Italian parsley or thyme and leeks or other vegetable scraps. Freeze the stock in ice cube trays for making pan sauces and in pint containers for making soups.

- 1 medium yellow onion, quartered
- 3 medium carrots, unpeeled, cut into 1-inch chunks
- 2 stalks celery, cut into 1-inch chunks
- 1 bay leaf
- 8 whole black peppercorns

Combine the onion, carrots, celery, bay leaf, and peppercorns in a large saucepan. Add 2 quarts of water and bring to a boil over medium heat. Reduce the heat, cover, and simmer for 30 minutes.

Strain into containers and refrigerate for up to 5 days or freeze for up to 1 month.

Salads & Sandwiches

Grilled Asparagus on Greens with Sun-Dried Cherries, Chèvre, and Toasted Pistachios

Roasted Vegetables with Manchego

Baby Spinach Salad with Pears, Toasted Walnuts, and Pecorino

Crab Salad with Cilantro and Chives

Curried Chicken Salad

French Lentil Salad

White Bean Salad with Olives and Frisée

Asian Cabbage Salad

Seaweed Salad

Bulgur Salad

Summer Vegetable Salad

Corn Salad with Bell Pepper and Cilantro

Corn Salad on Baby Greens with Avocado and Feta

Provençal Carrot Salad

When it comes to salads, I hear the same thing over and over: "I would eat more of them if I had the energy to make them." Though a beautiful, bountiful bowlful is more fun to sit down to than a sandwich, let's face it—putting something between two pieces of bread is much easier than washing, chopping, and dressing a salad.

This chapter doesn't have any salads that miraculously assemble themselves, but if you use shortcuts like prewashed and cut vegetables or canned organic beans, you may find yourself enjoying a salad in the same time it would take you to wait for your bread to toast. Speaking of bread, when what you really want is a sandwich, turn to the Feeling Food variations for the best ways to turn these healthful salads into satisfying sandwiches. You'll recognize them by the ⊞ symbol next to them.

And remember that adding just a cup of soup to your sandwich or salad meal will go a long way in helping your digestion (see page 47).

ABOUT SALAD DRESSINGS

The great intention behind eating a salad chock-full of vegetables can sometimes be undermined when it is drowned in salad dressing, even the healthiest kind. At Mothers & Menus, we recommend enjoying your salad with 1 tablespoon of dressing per serving, which is what you will find in the recipes that follow. This light touch really highlights the vegetables, but may not always be enough for all taste buds. Feel free to adjust the quantity of the salad dressing accordingly.

Grilled Asparagus on Greens with Sun-Dried Cherries, Chèvre, and Toasted Pistachios • SERVES 2 TO 4

Grilled vegetables lend great flavor to any meal or salad, but not everyone has the ability or inclination to fire up an outdoor grill. A stovetop grill pan is an easy, tasty, inexpensive way to enhance your cooking possibilities. Many grill pans flip over to a griddle on the other side, which is great for pancakes and French toast. If you do not have one, simply pan roast the asparagus on the stovetop in a heavy skillet, or oven roast them as directed on page 155.

 8 ounces pencil-thin asparagus, ends trimmed
 1 teaspoon olive oil
   Salt and freshly ground pepper
 6 cups loosely packed mixed greens
 4 ounces fresh goat cheese, plain, cracked pepper, or herb, cut into
   medallions or crumbled
 ¼ cup unsweetened dried cherries (not sour cherries)
 ¼ cup shelled pistachio nuts, toasted (see below)
 2 tablespoons Orange Vinaigrette (recipe follows), Balsamic Vinaigrette
   (page 73), or Sherry Vinaigrette (page 73)

Heat a grill pan over medium-high. Toss the asparagus with the olive oil and season with salt and pepper. Grill the asparagus until they are bright green and tender, rotating during cooking to cook on all sides, about 2 minutes. Remove to a plate and allow the asparagus to cool completely.

Divide the greens among 2 to 4 plates and fan out the asparagus on top of the greens. Arrange the goat cheese and cherries over the asparagus and sprinkle the pistachios on top. Drizzle with the vinaigrette.

To toast nuts: Preheat the oven to 350°F. Spread out the nuts on a sheet pan, and toast in the oven until golden brown, 5 to 12 mintues, depending on the type of nut. Cool completely before using. Store the nuts in an airtight container and keep in a cool dry place. They will keep for 3 weeks.

FEELING GREEN: Prepare the asparagus as directed. When cool, chop into 1-inch pieces. Divide the goat cheese into 2 portions, and spread onto 2 whole grain tortillas, wraps, or pitas. In a medium bowl, combine the greens, cherries, and pistachios with the Balsamic or Lemon-Dijon Vinaigrette (page 73 or 77). Mix well and place on or in the bread of choice.

FEELING FOOD: Prepare the asparagus as directed and set aside. Divide the goat cheese into 2 portions and spread onto 2 whole grain tortillas, wraps, or pitas. In a medium bowl, combine the greens, cherries, and pistachios with the Orange Vinaigrette. Mix well and place on or in the bread of choice. Enjoy with crispy Roasted Asparagus with Lemon (page 155) on the side.

FEELING FULL: Dried fruit is higher in sugar than its fresh counterpart, so replace the cherries in this salad with a fresh fruit such as chopped pear, apple, or orange sections. Reduce the amount of pistachios.

Orange Vinaigrette • MAKES 1 CUP

This subtly sweet dressing also works beautifully with baby spinach and walnuts.

$\frac{1}{3}$ cup fresh orange juice

1 teaspoon Dijon mustard

Salt and freshly ground pepper

$\frac{2}{3}$ cup extra virgin olive oil

1 tablespoon chopped fresh tarragon, optional

1 tablespoon chopped fresh chives

Whisk together the orange juice, mustard, and salt and pepper to taste. Whisk in the olive oil. When ready to serve, whisk in the fresh herbs. The vinaigrette will keep for 1 week in the refrigerator.

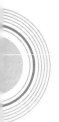

Roasted Vegetables with Manchego • SERVES 2 TO 4

I make this salad often, especially when I'm having company. It is easy to pull together and absolutely beautiful to behold. Use your creativity to arrange vegetables for maximum effect. Add some Bruschetta or Crostini (page 102) with your favorite toppings for an elegant, light summer meal.

6 cups loosely packed mixed baby greens, such as mesclun, baby spinach, baby arugula, or a combination

2 cups roasted vegetables (see pages 155 to 159), such as asparagus, mushrooms, and tomatoes

4 ounces Manchego or another hard cheese, sliced ¼ inch thick

½ cup cherry or grape tomatoes, halved

Fresh basil or tarragon leaves for garnish, optional

2 tablespoons Balsamic Vinaigrette (recipe follows)

Divide the greens among 2 to 4 plates. Arrange the roasted vegetables on top, fanning out longer shapes (such as asparagus) and laying smaller vegetables (such as mushrooms) at the base of the fan.

Arrange the Manchego slices over the vegetables and top the salad with cherry tomatoes and basil. Drizzle with the vinaigrette and serve immediately.

FEELING GREEN: Choose asparagus and mushrooms for your vegetables; a gentle, creamy cheese, such as fresh goat cheese; and reduce the greens to whatever you can handle.

FEELING FOOD: Use Lemon-Dijon Vinaigrette (page 77) instead of Balsamic, and spread over lightly toasted sourdough bread. Layer on the cheese, greens, and roasted vegetables.

FEELING FULL: Reduce the cheese by half and enjoy!

Balsamic Vinaigrette • MAKES 1 CUP

This dressing is so smooth and thick, it almost seems creamy. Use a good-quality balsamic vinegar for a vinaigrette that is flavorful, but not overly sweet.

⅓ cup balsamic vinegar
1 small shallot, minced
1 tablespoon Dijon mustard
  Salt and freshly ground pepper
⅔ cup extra-virgin olive oil

In a small bowl, whisk together the vinegar, shallot, mustard, and salt and pepper to taste in a small bowl or blend in a blender. Add the oil in a slow, steady trickle and continue whisking or blending until smooth. The dressing will keep for 2 weeks in the refrigerator.

SHERRY VINAIGRETTE: Substitute ¼ cup of sherry vinegar and 1 teaspoon of honey for the balsamic vinegar. Proceed as directed.

CHAMPAGNE AND HERB VINAIGRETTE: Substitute ¼ cup of champagne vinegar for the balsamic. Add 1 tablespoon of chopped fresh tarragon (or other fresh herbs) before serving.

 ABOUT BALSAMIC

Real balsamic vinegar can only be produced in the regions of Modena and Reggio in Italy. In the Middle Ages it was used as a miracle cure. These days, balsamic vinegar is reported to improve metabolism, strengthen bones, and fight anemia and fatigue. It has acquired a reputation on pregnancy blogs as a labor inducer and a relief for morning sickness when drunk from a shot glass.

Baby Spinach Salad with Pears, Toasted Walnuts, and Pecorino • SERVES 2

It is hard to believe that just forty years ago, spinach was most commonly consumed in the United States from a can (think Popeye). While fresh baby spinach is now readily available all year long, this salad is perfect in late fall and early winter, when pears are at their best.

4 cups loosely packed baby spinach leaves

1 medium pear, such as Bosc or Bartlett

4 ounces hard pecorino cheese, crumbled (¼ cup)

¼ cup walnuts, toasted (see page 70)

2 tablespoons Sherry Vinaigrette (page 73)

Divide the spinach between 2 plates. Cut the pear in half. Remove the core and stem with a small knife, and cut the pears lengthwise into ½-inch-thick slices. Fan out the pear slices on top of the spinach.

Sprinkle the cheese and walnuts over the pear, and drizzle each serving with 1 tablespoon of Sherry Vinaigrette. Serve immediately.

FEELING GREEN: When you are feeling green, raw green vegetables often drop to the bottom of the what-I-want-to-eat list. Try wilting the greens instead. Put the spinach in a bowl. Heat 3 tablespoons of olive oil and ½ teaspoon of salt in a small pan over high heat until nearly smoking. Turn off the heat, pour the hot oil over the spinach, and toss to coat. Divide between 2 plates, and top with the pear, cheese, and nuts, but do not add the sherry vinaigrette. Instead, spritz liberally with fresh lemon juice.

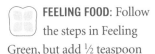 **FEELING FOOD**: Follow the steps in Feeling Green, but add ½ teaspoon of Dijon mustard to the oil and salt prior to heating. Pack all of the salad ingredients into a whole wheat pita pocket for a healthy, warm, and comforting meal.

FEELING FULL: Replace the cheese with 4 ounces of grilled chicken, which will work well with the fruit and nuts.

Crab Salad with Cilantro and Chives • SERVES 3 TO 4

This simple salad highlights best-quality fresh or pasteurized crabmeat (don't used canned). Serve with a mixed green salad, sliced avocado, or crisp steamed vegetables for an extra special lunch or summer supper.

1 pound lump crabmeat, picked over to remove any cartilage or shell
2 stalks celery, finely chopped
2 tablespoons chopped fresh cilantro
1 tablespoon chopped fresh chives
3 tablespoons mayonnaise, or to taste
1 tablespoon fresh lime juice
   Pinch of cayenne pepper, optional
   Salt and freshly ground pepper

In a small bowl, toss the crabmeat, celery, cilantro, and chives with the mayonnaise, lime juice, cayenne, and salt and pepper to taste. The salad will keep for up to 1 day in the refrigerator.

FEELING GREEN: Right now, crab probably is not for you, regardless of the variation. If you're in the mood for some seafood, try the Feeling Green version of the Tuna Salad (page 101).

FEELING FOOD: Spread a soft challah or brioche roll with mayonnaise and layer with lettuce and tomato before piling on the crab salad.

FEELING FULL: Reduce the mayonnaise to 1 tablespoon. Enjoy a scoop of the salad over your favorite mixed greens, seasoned with Lemon-Dijon Vinaigrette (page 77).

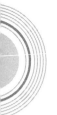

Curried Chicken Salad • SERVES 2

Even people who are not big curry fans love this chicken salad, possibly because the curry is mixed into mayonnaise, which mellows it. This is a great way to jazz up leftover cooked chicken, especially after making Chicken Stock (page 66). Serve this salad as is, between two slices of bread, or over greens with a dollop of chutney to elevate this classic to a new experience.

1 teaspoon curry powder
2 tablespoons mayonnaise
  Spritz of lime juice
2 cups diced cooked chicken
½ cup diced celery
1 teaspoon chopped scallion, green part only
  Salt and freshly ground pepper

If you have time, lightly toast the curry powder in a small skillet over medium heat to release the flavor, about 1 minute. Otherwise, use straight from the jar. Transfer to a bowl and stir in the mayonnaise and lime juice.

Stir in the chicken, celery, and scallions and season to taste with salt and pepper. The salad will keep for up to 3 days in the refrigerator.

Express: Stock your freezer with organic, precooked, diced chicken, such as Eberly's. Freshly prepared is always preferable, but having some on hand will take you far in terms of preparing a quick chicken salad, and it's a good add-in to stir-fries such as Stir-Fried Vegetables with Coconut Curry Sauce (page 137).

FEELING GREEN: Omit the curry powder, mayonnaise, lime juice, and scallions. Season the chicken with Lemon-Dijon Vinaigrette (recipe follows) and a good sprinkle of parsley, which can help minimize nausea.

FEELING FOOD: Spread a whole grain wrap with mayonnaise or chutney, and top with the chicken salad and some lettuce and tomato slices.

FEELING FULL: Reduce the mayonnaise to 1 tablespoon and add toasted curry powder to taste. Please, do not go low-fat on the mayonnaise; it is full of additives and not nearly as satiating. Enjoy the salad over a bed of mesclun or baby greens.

Lemon-Dijon Vinaigrette • MAKES 1 CUP

This light, bright dressing is great on niçoise salads, baby spinach, and steamed vegetables and is perfect for anyone who is sensitive to vinegar.

1/3 cup fresh lemon juice

1 tablespoon Dijon mustard

1 small shallot, minced

Salt and freshly ground pepper

2/3 cup extra-virgin olive oil

Whisk together the lemon juice, mustard, shallot, and salt and pepper to taste. Whisk in the oil. The dressing will keep for 2 weeks in the refrigerator.

French Lentil Salad • SERVES 4

This protein-packed salad is easy to digest and beautiful to behold with its tiny flecks of carrot, celery, tomato, and herbs. Use small green or gray French lentils for this dish; they hold their shape and texture better than their larger counterparts.

1 cup French lentils
1 bay leaf
1 clove garlic
1 medium carrot, peeled and finely chopped
1 stalk celery, finely chopped
1 medium plum tomato, seeded and finely chopped
1 tablespoon chopped fresh Italian parsley
1 tablespoon chopped fresh chives
1½ tablespoons fresh lemon juice
¼ cup extra-virgin olive oil
   Salt and freshly ground pepper

Combine the lentils, bay leaf, and garlic in a medium saucepan and add enough water to cover by 1 inch. Bring to a boil, reduce the heat to medium-low, and cook until the lentils are firm but tender, about 15 minutes. Drain and let cool. Discard the bay leaf and garlic.

In a medium bowl, combine the lentils with the carrot, celery, tomato, parsley, chives, lemon juice, and olive oil. Season to taste with salt and pepper. The salad will keep for up to 3 days in the refrigerator.

FEELING GREEN: This dish is great when you are feeling green because the lentils are easy to digest, as are the finely chopped vegetables. If you are very queasy, skip the chives. When seasoning to taste, try adding more lemon.

FEELING FOOD: Sprinkle some goat cheese over this salad and enjoy it with a hunk of fresh, crusty baguette.

FEELING FULL: No adaptation necessary! This high-protein, low-fat, veggie-filled salad is delicious, nutritious, and will keep you full without feeling stuffed.

White Bean Salad with Olives and Frisée • SERVES 3 TO 4

Every Mediterranean country seems to have a version of this delicious salad. In Turkey, cooked white beans are mixed with raw onions and hard-boiled eggs. In France, picholine olives and fresh rosemary are commonly paired with the beans. Lebanon and Italy have their own popular versions as well. Here is a combination that brings together maximum ease, nutrition, and, of course, flavor.

1 (15-ounce) can small white beans, rinsed and drained
½ cup sliced pitted black cerignola or other large, firm olives
1 stalk celery, finely chopped
1 tablespoon chopped fresh Italian parsley
1 tablespoon fresh lemon juice
1 small clove garlic, minced
2 tablespoons extra-virgin olive oil
Salt and freshly ground pepper
4 cups torn frisée lettuce (about 1 medium head)

In a medium bowl, combine the beans, olives, celery, and parsley.

In a small bowl, whisk together the lemon juice, garlic, and olive oil. Stir gently into the beans. Season to taste with salt and pepper. At this point, the salad can be refrigerated for up to 1 day.

To serve, gently toss the frisée leaves with the bean salad and divide among 4 salad plates.

In a pinch: If frisée is unavailable, baby arugula, radicchio, or even romaine makes a great alternative.

FEELING GREEN: Some say that mashed beans are easier to digest because the enzymes are broken down. With that in mind, you might want to try out the White Bean Dip with Crudités (page 95).

FEELING FOOD: Prepare as directed. Add some crumbled feta cheese, and enjoy your portion on fresh lavash (a soft, thin flatbread of Armenian origin) or, alternatively, in a whole wheat pita.

FEELING FULL: Turn this salad into a high-protein meal by adding hard-boiled eggs, steamed shrimp, or canned salmon, and some steamed green beans or grilled asparagus.

Asian Cabbage Salad • SERVES 4 TO 6

This crunchy, crispy, juicy, and highly flavorful salad is a fantastic and refreshing alternative to traditional coleslaw. Edamame, sesame oil, rice vinegar, sambal (see opposite), and black sesame seeds are available in many supermarkets, in Asian markets, and in health food stores.

  1 (12-ounce) package frozen shelled edamame
½ head red cabbage, finely shredded (4 cups)
½ head green or napa cabbage, finely shredded (4 cups)
  2 medium carrots, finely shredded (2 cups)
  4 scallions, green and white parts, finely chopped
  2 tablespoons toasted sesame oil
¾ cup seasoned rice vinegar
  1 tablespoon peeled and grated fresh ginger
  1 teaspoon sambal or another ground chile paste, optional
  2 tablespoons black sesame seeds
    Fresh cilantro leaves for garnish

Cook the edamame according to the package directions, drain, and set aside to cool.

In a large bowl, combine the edamame, red and green cabbages, carrots, and scallions. In a small bowl, whisk together the oil, vinegar, ginger, and sambal, if using. Pour the dressing over the slaw, mix well, and refrigerate for at least 2 hours or overnight, so that the flavors can meld.

Serve garnished with the sesame seeds and cilantro.

ABOUT SAMBAL

Sambal is a delicious, spicy paste made up of a variety of peppers, most often chile peppers. It is a condiment used in Indonesia, Malaysia, Singapore, and Sri Lanka. Look for sambal in the Asian section of your supermarket. If you can't find it, try a dash of hot chile sauce instead.

FEELING GREEN: When you are feeling green, foods that are known to cause bloating may aggravate the nausea, and cabbage is one of those foods. So replace the cabbage with a total of 1 pound carrots, grated, for an Asian carrot slaw. Omit the scallions and the sambal. Taste the sesame seeds prior to serving to see if you enjoy them.

FEELING FOOD: This tasty salad may become your new comfort slaw, but if you are yearning for traditional coleslaw, try this: Skip the edamame, sesame oil, rice vinegar, ginger, sambal, sesame seeds, and cilantro. Instead, whisk together 2 tablespoons of cider vinegar with ¾ cup of mayonnaise and pour the mixture over the cabbage and carrots. Now add a handful of raisins and ¼ cup unsweetened shredded coconut and mix well. Taste and add some salt, if needed, to balance the flavors.

FEELING FULL: This fiber-, calcium-, and vitamin C–rich salad does not need any fine-tuning. It is a flavorful, nutritious, low-calorie snack; top it with some tofu to turn it into a high-protein entree.

LEGEND HAS IT . . .

Cabbage has been used since ancient times as a remedy for engorgement. Place thoroughly washed cabbage leaves, chilled or not, in your bra. This will not only help to relieve engorgement, but may also start to reduce your milk supply. So use only as needed, and change every 2 to 3 hours.

Seaweed Salad • SERVES 4

Seaweed, such as wakame, is a veritable superfood. It is reputed to enhance immune function, aid in digestion, and provide relief from aches and pains. It is abundantly high in fiber, iron, and calcium. In fact, wakame contains over twice the amount of calcium found in milk. It's also incredibly satisfying and toothsome and pairs exceptionally well with Asian flavors, as in this refreshing salad. You can find dried wakame, as well as daikon radish, in many supermarkets and in any Asian specialty store.

- ½ cup dried wakame seaweed, preferably with short tips
- 1 medium carrot, peeled and shredded
- 1 small daikon radish, peeled and shredded (½ cup)
- 2 scallions, white and green parts, thinly sliced
- 2 tablespoons seasoned rice vinegar
- 2 teaspoons toasted sesame oil
- Pinch of cayenne pepper, optional
- Salt and freshly ground pepper
- 1 tablespoon white sesame seeds

Bring 2 cups of water to a boil over high heat. Put the wakame in a medium heat-proof bowl and pour the water on top. Let the wakame soak for 15 minutes. Drain and pat the wakame dry and cut into bite-size pieces. Wipe the bowl dry. Return the wakame to the bowl and add the carrot, daikon, scallions, vinegar, oil, cayenne, and salt and pepper to taste. Toss well.

Let the salad sit for at least 30 minutes at room temperature or up to 1 day in the refrigerator before serving. Garnish with sesame seeds when you are ready to serve.

FEELING GREEN: Unless you are a huge fan of seaweed, this salad may make you greener. But if you are willing to give it a shot, try the Feeling Food version.

FEELING FOOD: Soak and drain the wakame as indicated and stir in the carrot, daikon, scallions, and one 12-ounce package of frozen shelled edamame, cooked according to the package directions and drained. Omit the vinegar and sesame oil and instead prepare Tahini Dressing (page 94). Season the salad with some of the dressing and enjoy over a serving of Sesame Lotus Root Soba Noodles (page 167).

FEELING FULL: This powerful salad will revitalize your digestive system and bring you a bevy of other benefits, including the naturally occurring fat-burning compound found in wakame. For a healthy entree, serve it with a cup of steamed brown rice, sautéed kale, and a dollop of Carrot-Ginger Dressing (recipe follows).

Carrot-Ginger Dressing • MAKES ABOUT 1 CUP

Bright in flavor and low in fat, this brilliant orange dressing pairs perfectly with summer salads, grilled dishes, and just about any kind of tofu. Keep in mind that it has a distinctive flavor and will not serve as an all-purpose everyday vinaigrette unless you are eating a lot of Asian-inspired food. Because this dressing is made predominantly of raw carrots, it will not keep as long as vinaigrettes with a dominant vinegar base.

> 1 cup peeled and grated carrots (about 2 medium to small carrots)
> 2 tablespoons peeled and grated fresh ginger
> 2 tablespoons seasoned rice vinegar
> 1 tablespoon toasted sesame oil
> 1½ teaspoons soy sauce
> Freshly ground pepper
> Finely chopped scallions, white and green parts, for garnish, optional

Combine the carrots, ginger, vinegar, oil, soy sauce, and ⅓ cup of cold water in a blender. Season with a pinch of pepper and blend until smooth. If the dressing is too thick to pour out of the blender, add additional water, 1 tablespoon at a time. The dressing will keep for up to 3 days in the refrigerator. Garnish the salad with scallions, if desired.

Bulgur Salad • SERVES 4

A variation on traditional tabouli, this recipe incorporates fresh corn, Kirby cucumbers, and basil leaves, which add flavor and crunch to the salad. A sprinkling of crumbled feta or ricotta salata adds extra nutrients, but you can substitute cooked chickpeas for a high-protein vegan dish.

1 cup medium-grind bulgur
½ teaspoon salt
1 cup fresh or frozen corn kernels (about 2 ears)
4 plum tomatoes, seeded and diced
2 Kirby cucumbers, diced
1 cup fresh Italian parsley leaves, chopped
6 scallions, white and green parts, finely chopped
1 cup fresh mint leaves, finely chopped
1 cup fresh basil leaves, thinly sliced
⅓ cup extra-virgin olive oil
⅓ cup fresh lemon juice
   Salt and freshly ground pepper
4 ounces feta or ricotta salata cheese, crumbled (½ cup)

Bring 2 cups of water to a boil over high heat. Put the bulgur and salt in a heat-proof medium bowl, pour in the water, and cover with plastic wrap or a plate. Let it sit until all the water is absorbed, about 30 minutes. Drain if needed and cool completely before using.

Bring 1 or 2 inches of water to a boil in the bottom of a steamer or a medium pot fitted with a steamer insert. Add the corn, cover the steamer, and steam until the corn is tender, about 5 minutes.

Add the corn, tomatoes, cucumber, parsley, scallions, mint, and basil to the bulgur. Drizzle the olive oil and lemon juice over the top, season with salt and pepper, and toss well. Top with the crumbled feta. The salad will keep for 2 days in the refrigerator.

FEELING GREEN: Parsley and mint are two herbs that have been used for centuries to ward off nausea. Reduce the tomatoes from 4 to 2 and omit the scallions. Prepare as directed.

FEELING FOOD: Stuff this salad into a whole wheat pita for a delicious sandwich.

FEELING FULL: While bulgur is a terrific source of magnesium and fiber and a whole grain, it is essentially a wheat product. Substitute 2 cups steamed quinoa (see page 173) for the bulgur.

Summer Vegetable Salad • SERVES 4 TO 6

This cheerful bowl of greens with splashes of orange, white, and red doubles as a salad entree or side vegetable. You can substitute your favorite vinaigrette for the lemon and olive oil, but always wait until serving to dress the vegetables; otherwise they will lose their bright color because of the acid in the dressing.

4 ounces green beans, trimmed and cut on the bias into 1-inch pieces
4 ounces sugar snap or snow peas, cut on the bias in half
4 ounces medium asparagus, stems removed, cut on the bias into 1-inch pieces
2 Kirby cucumbers, cut in half lengthwise and sliced ¼ inch thick
1 medium carrot, cut in half lengthwise and thinly sliced
½ cup cherry or grape tomatoes, cut in half
1 tablespoon chopped fresh chives
1 tablespoon chopped fresh herbs, such as dill, basil, tarragon, or mint
3 tablespoons extra-virgin olive oil
1 tablespoon fresh lemon juice
Salt and freshly ground pepper

Bring 2 quarts of salted water to a boil over high heat. Have ready a large bowl filled halfway with ice water. Add the green beans, peas, and asparagus to the boiling water, return to a boil, and cook the vegetables for 1 minute. They should be bright green. Drain and transfer to the ice water to stop the cooking. Once cool, drain well.

In a medium bowl, toss the cooked vegetables, the cucumbers, carrot, tomatoes, chives, and herbs. At this point, the salad can be refrigerated for up to 8 hours.

To serve, toss the salad with the olive oil, lemon juice, and salt and pepper to taste.

FEELING GREEN: When the thought of eating a raw salad makes you greener, this salad, with its cooked mild vegetables and lemon dressing, may become your salad of choice. Skip the tomatoes and chives, and opt for mint as your herb.

FEELING FOOD: Skip the carrot and the chives and prepare as directed. Smear Classic Hummus (page 92) or White Bean Dip (page 95) on 2 slices of dense, artisanal whole grain bread. Scoop the salad onto the bread and enjoy a crunchy, creamy sandwich combination.

FEELING FULL: With the salad's seasonal vegetables and fresh herbs and lemon juice, olive oil will not be missed, so feel free to do without.

Corn Salad with Bell Pepper and Cilantro • MAKES 4 CUPS

Fresh corn is best for this salad, which is crunchy, slightly spicy, and simply delicious. Serve with grilled or seared fish or chicken, or as part of a bright summer entree salad (see Corn Salad on Baby Greens with Avocado and Feta, opposite).

6 ears corn, husks and silk removed (3 cups)
1 small red bell pepper, seeded and finely diced
1 small jalapeño, seeded and minced
2 scallions, green part only, finely chopped
¼ cup chopped fresh cilantro
2 tablespoons fresh lime juice
2 tablespoons extra-virgin olive oil
Salt and freshly ground pepper

Bring 1 or 2 inches of water to a boil in the bottom of a steamer or a medium pot fitted with a steamer insert. Add the corn, cover the steamer, and steam until the corn is tender, about 7 minutes. Rinse under cold running water to stop the cooking.

With a very sharp knife, cut the kernels from cobs into a medium bowl. Add the bell pepper, jalapeño, scallions, cilantro, lime juice, olive oil, and salt and pepper to taste and toss well. The salad will keep for up to 1 day in the refrigerator.

In a pinch: Chives are a wonderful alternative to scallions, and fresh basil can replace the cilantro. Baby tomatoes, halved, or seeded and diced plum or beefsteak tomatoes can be substituted for the red pepper. Replace fresh corn with frozen, steam for just 5 minutes. In a real pinch, use canned.

FEELING GREEN: Replace the bell pepper with a tomato. Skip the jalapeño and scallions, and follow the recipe as directed.

FEELING FOOD: Crumbled feta cheese and creamy avocado turn this corn salad into a creamy, crunchy treat. Check out the Feeling Food variation opposite for a sandwich suggestion.

FEELING FULL: This delicious salad will satisfy your sweet tooth and give you energy to spare. Serve over baby arugula for an additional crunch.

Corn Salad on Baby Greens with Avocado and Feta • SERVES 2 TO 4

Sweet, crunchy, creamy, and green, this salad is also packed with nutrients. Be sure to pick a ripe but firm avocado and very fresh corn for optimal results.

- 1 large Hass avocado
- ½ lime
- 6 cups loosely packed baby greens or mesclun
- ½ recipe Corn Salad with Bell Pepper and Cilantro (opposite)
- 1 plum tomato, cut into 8 wedges
- 4 ounces Greek feta cheese, crumbled (½ cup)
- 1 tablespoon fresh lime juice
- 2 tablespoons extra-virgin olive oil
- Salt and freshly ground pepper

Cut the avocado in half lengthwise and remove the pit. Scoop out the flesh from each skin in 1 piece. Slice each half lengthwise into 5 to 7 segments. Fan out slightly and spritz with lime juice.

Divide the greens among 2 to 4 plates. Top with avocado and some corn salad. Arrange the tomato wedges alongside the corn and top with feta. Sprinkle each salad with lime juice, olive oil, and salt and pepper to taste. Serve immediately.

FEELING GREEN: Enjoy the Feeling Green variation of the corn salad opposite and add the cheese and lime-spritzed avocado. Skip the greens, tomato, and olive oil. Season to taste.

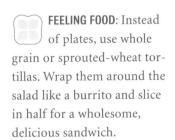 **FEELING FOOD**: Instead of plates, use whole grain or sprouted-wheat tortillas. Wrap them around the salad like a burrito and slice in half for a wholesome, delicious sandwich.

FEELING FULL: For a summer dinner, replace the feta with steamed shrimp, broiled fish, or grilled chicken.

LEGEND HAS IT . . .

At a time when pregnancy was believed to be controlled by spirits, women's birth control strategies were passed down secretly to mothers who felt they already had too many children. One prescribed method was turning a spinning wheel backward at midnight. Another was throwing corn kernels into a well at a magical hour.

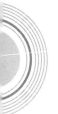

Provençal Carrot Salad • SERVES 4

A simple classic from the south of France, this dish features sweet, juicy, crisp carrots, simply seasoned. It is often served alongside other salads, or as a palate-cleansing side dish for highly seasoned entrees. Keep traveling south, and you will end up in Morocco, where a sweet take on this salad is popular. See the Feeling Green and Feeling Food variations.

1 pound carrots, peeled and grated
3 tablespoons extra-virgin olive oil
1 tablespoon fresh lemon juice
   Salt and freshly ground pepper
2 tablespoons chopped fresh Italian parsley
1 tablespoon chopped fresh mint

In a medium bowl, toss the carrots with the olive oil and lemon juice. Season to taste with salt and pepper. At this point, the salad can be refrigerated for several hours.

To serve, gently toss in the parsley and mint.

FEELING GREEN: Add 1 tablespoon of lemon juice, ¾ teaspoon of peeled and grated fresh ginger, and ½ teaspoon of ground cinnamon. Prepare as directed and see if you can add just a bit more mint to leverage its soothing properties.

FEELING FOOD: Dissolve 2 tablespoons of honey into ¼ cup of lemon juice and omit the olive oil. Add to the carrots along with ¼ teaspoon of ground cinnamon and ½ cup of golden raisins.

FEELING FULL: Reduce the olive oil to 2 teaspoons and add ½ teaspoon of flax seed oil to power up the nutrients of this already healthy salad.

REAL WORLD

With a kitchen under renovation, I have no access to the oven, and with the heat we are having, I am not inclined to go there anyway. This carrot salad was such an easy, refreshing pick-me-up! I loved the crunchy texture and especially the parsley and mint combo, which I hadn't thought to try before. My son, Luca, almost two, just loved this dish, but asked for more carrots in his portion, since it's one of his favorite vegetables.

Lisa Arezzi, New York, NY

Snacks

So many of us were raised to believe that snacking is something that we should try to avoid, when in fact, daylong grazing is an excellent way to stabilize your blood sugar, keep you energized, stave away cravings, and keep nausea at bay. So why the controversy? It has more to do with *what* we call a snack.

Instead of thinking of snacks as empty-calorie foods with little or no nutritive value, such as pretzels and cookies, think of them as mini-meals: a cup of soup, half a sandwich, a piece of fruit and a handful of nuts, White Bean Dip with Crudités (page 95). And check out the Desserts chapter to fuel up on a Jam Dot Cookie (page 177) or an Ultra-Energy Bar (page 180).

The trick to great snacking is being prepared. When you run out of the house with nothing in your bag, you often end up eating something you otherwise wouldn't, or you end up starving, leading you to eat a heavier wish-I-hadn't meal. Try this instead: When you bring home the groceries, fill sandwich baggies with baby carrots, cherry tomatoes, nuts, grapes, cubed cheese, and whole grain crackers—anything that can make a quick and easy on-the-go snack. Now, just remember to grab a baggie before you head out the door. This is a great thing to practice while you are pregnant; once you have kids, you will always need to pack some sort of snack for them when you leave the house. You never know where you'll be—in the car, waiting in line, at the doctor's office, or at the playground—when a little nibble will make the difference between a cranky kid and a happy camper.

THAT'S ENTERTAINMENT

Think of this chapter as your guide to entertaining as well. Whether you are hosting a party or bringing a dish to one, the recipes in this chapter will allow you to spend minimum time for maximum results. Look for "That's Entertainment" tips along the way.

Classic Hummus • MAKES 2 CUPS

Chickpeas are an excellent source of protein, fiber, and folate; so eat up! Hummus *is the Arabic and Hebrew name for "chickpea," but it is better known as a tasty, creamy dip. Try it with crudités or pita chips—or as a vegetarian sandwich filler with roasted or raw vegetables.*

1 (15-ounce) can chickpeas, rinsed and drained
6 tablespoons fresh lemon juice
1 clove garlic
3 tablespoons tahini paste (see page 94)
    Salt and freshly ground pepper
1 tablespoon extra-virgin olive oil, optional
1 tablespoon chopped fresh Italian parsley
    Paprika for garnish

Puree the chickpeas, lemon juice, garlic, and tahini in a food processor, adding up to ¼ cup of cold water to obtain a creamy consistency. Season with salt and pepper to taste.

Mound on a small serving plate and flatten with the back of a tablespoon. Drizzle with the olive oil and sprinkle with the parsley and paprika. Hummus will keep for several days, refrigerated.

REAL WORLD

Having lived in Israel for a number of years, both my husband and I are big hummus fans. I had been wanting to make it at home, but could not find a good, easy recipe, and always opted for the convenient store-bought ones. But this was so easy! The whole thing took 10 minutes. I particularly enjoyed the roasted garlic [see Feeling Green], which gave it a wonderful flavor. I spread some in a pita for Lani, four, to try and was thrilled to get an okay from her!

Yasmin Ben-Dror, Fairlawn, NJ

FEELING GREEN: Make hummus with roasted garlic, eliminating the raw garlic, which can be difficult to digest. Follow the recipe for Classic Hummus, substituting 3 roasted garlic cloves (see page 97) for the raw. Spread in a warmed pita and add sliced cucumbers.

FEELING FOOD: Make baba ghanoush, a cousin of hummus, which includes roasted eggplant in the mix for an even heartier version. Preheat the oven to 400°F. Slice a large eggplant in half and roast, face up, on a baking sheet, until soft and browned, about 45 minutes. Allow to cool. Scoop out the inside of the eggplant and add to the food processor along with the chickpeas, lemon juice, garlic, and water. Puree and season with salt and pepper. Spread out on a small plate, creating a well in the middle. Fill with Tahini Dressing (page 94), and mop everything up with warm, soft pita bread. Makes 3 cups.

FEELING FULL: Make a Mediterranean lemon and herb chickpea spread without the tahini for a lighter result. Sauté 2 sliced shallots and 1 sliced clove garlic in 2 tablespoons of olive oil until soft, but not brown, 3 to 5 minutes. Stir in ¼ cup of chopped fresh basil and 1 tablespoon of chopped fresh Italian parsley. Puree in a food processor with the chickpeas, ⅓ cup of fresh lemon juice, salt and pepper to taste, and enough water to make a smooth paste. Enjoy over a salad of diced cucumber, tomato, scallion, and parsley dressed with olive oil and lemon juice.

ABOUT HUMMUS

Because of its long history (more than three thousand years), no one is clear about the origins of hummus, though many cultures claim it as their own. Some say that connoisseurs can accurately identify a Middle Easterner's family lineage based on his or her recipe for hummus. For example, it is said that religious families load their hummus with garlic, ostensibly as a means of keeping their young men and women separated (keep this in mind for when your baby becomes a teenager).

Tahini Dressing • MAKES ABOUT 1 CUP

Tahini is a thick paste made of ground sesame seeds, which are an excellent source of copper, calcium, magnesium, iron phosphorous, and vitamin B1. Because of tahini's strong, nutty essence, just a little of the paste contributes a rich flavor. Look for it in health food stores or Middle Eastern specialty stores. In Israel, tahini dressing, called tehina, *is as common as ketchup in the U.S. Used in sandwiches, on salads, with vegetables, over falafel, and with hummus, this dressing's versatility, taste, and ease of preparation make it a must-have. The scallions and parsley in this recipe take tahini's boring beige to a beautiful, bright green.*

½ cup tahini paste
2 tablespoons fresh lemon juice
1 tablespoon chopped scallion, green and white parts
1 clove garlic
2 tablespoons chopped fresh Italian parsley
½ teaspoon salt
Pinch of freshly ground pepper

Combine the tahini paste, ⅔ cup water, the lemon juice, scallion, garlic, parsley, salt, and pepper in a blender and blend on high speed until smooth. Store in the refrigerator for up to 5 days.

Express: Sesame seeds are also used to make a delicious Middle Eastern treat called halva. For a quick and healthy halvalike treat, spread tahini paste (just the paste, not the dressing) on your choice of toast and drizzle with some honey. Yum!

THAT'S ENTERTAINMENT | Middle-Eastern Delight

Make: A hummus recipe of choice, Tahini Dressing (above), and a Bulgur Salad (page 84).

Buy: Greek or Tunisian olives, stuffed grape leaves from the deli or (yes, I'll say it) canned; Mediterranean yogurt or cheese, such as Greek tzaziki or Lebanese labaneh; artichoke hearts; roasted red peppers; white and whole wheat pita bread; lemons; lemonade; and fresh mint.

To serve: Create a platter with the bowls of hummus, grape leaves, cheese, olives, artichoke hearts, and roasted peppers. Fill the spaces around and in between the bowls with quartered pitas (put some extra on the side). Decorate with a drizzle of olive oil and lemon wedges.

To drink: Pour lemonade into a pitcher and add branches of mint.

White Bean Dip with Crudités • SERVES 4 TO 6

In Italy, you will find white bean purees in the northern regions, while chickpeas are more common to the south, where the North African influence is much stronger. White bean dip is traditionally served with raw vegetables, which contain enzymes to aid with digestion. White bean dip is also great for spreading on bread or crackers and for using as a sandwich filling with grilled vegetables or lettuce, tomato, and sprouts.

2 tablespoons extra-virgin olive oil
1 small shallot, thinly sliced
2 cloves garlic, minced
1 teaspoon chopped fresh rosemary
1 teaspoon chopped fresh thyme
1 (15-ounce) can white beans, rinsed and drained
  Juice of 1 lemon
  Salt and freshly ground pepper
4 to 6 cups assorted vegetables, such as carrots, celery, or cucumber sticks; radishes; snow or snap peas; cherry tomatoes; asparagus; green beans; or bell peppers strips

In a small skillet, heat the olive oil over medium heat. Add the shallot and garlic and cook until soft, but not browned, about 5 minutes. Add the rosemary and thyme, cook for 1 minute, and transfer the mixture to the bowl of a food processor. Add the beans and lemon juice and puree, adding enough cold water to make a creamy paste. Season with salt and pepper to taste. The dip can be stored in an airtight container in the refrigerator for up to 5 days. Serve the dip in a small bowl on a platter filled with the vegetables.

FEELING GREEN: Add an extra spritz of lemon to this creamy, nutritious spread and try it on your favorite cracker.

FEELING FOOD: Dollop this on Crostini (page 102) spread with Tapenade (page 103) or drizzle with olive oil for a tasty treat.

FEELING FULL: Put a scoop of the bean dip on greens such as frisée, raddichio, or endive and add some olives and chopped celery for a delicious, filling salad.

Salsa Cruda • MAKES ABOUT 2 CUPS

Tomatoes are one of those great foods that are easy to love, easy to enjoy, and also really good for you—chock-full of antioxidants, lycopene, and vitamins. This homemade salsa is yet another fun way to eat tomatoes, but beware; once you try it out, you may never go back to store-bought. Fortunately, this salsa is so easy to make that you might not even care.

Double the recipe if you're feeding a crowd—you can even let a food processor do the chopping for you; just don't go overboard or you'll be making soup.

3 medium tomatoes, seeded and finely chopped
½ small red onion, finely chopped
1 jalapeño, seeded and finely chopped
2 tablespoons extra-virgin olive oil
½ cup chopped fresh cilantro
Juice of 1 lime
Salt and freshly ground pepper

Combine the tomatoes, onion, jalapeño, oil, cilantro, and lime juice in a large bowl. Season with salt and pepper and mix well. This will keep in the refrigerator for up to 2 days.

FEELING GREEN: This salsa, with its layers of flavors and bite, is probably not for you. Try Grilled Tomato Salsa (opposite). The smoother texture and the mellow flavors of the grilled vegetables may be easier to digest.

FEELING FOOD: Scoop up this salsa and Creamy Guacamole (page 98) with baked tortilla chips.

FEELING FULL: This salsa is a terrific, low-fat way to liven up a plate of grilled fish, chicken, beef, or tofu.

Grilled Tomato Salsa • MAKES 2 CUPS

Grilling the vegetables, roasting the garlic, and popping the cloves out of their skins takes much more time than a typical salsa—but there is nothing typical about this salsa. Its smoky, roasted flavors make it a hit at any party and an excellent salsa for any grilled dish. It also keeps well in the fridge for up to a week. All told, well worth the effort.

3	medium beefsteak tomatoes
	Olive oil for coating vegetables
½	medium red onion, cut into ½-inch-thick slices
2	cloves roasted garlic (see below)
½	canned chipotle chile, seeded and chopped
1½	teaspoons chopped fresh oregano
	Salt and freshly ground pepper

Heat a grill pan over medium-high heat.

Coat the tomatoes lightly with oil and set on the grill pan. Brush the onion slices with oil, being careful not to break them into rings, and place alongside the tomatoes. Grill the vegetables until well browned on all sides, about 10 minutes. Remove to a large mixing bowl and set aside to cool. Add the garlic, chipotle chile, and oregano and season with salt and pepper. Puree in a blender until the vegetables are blended but the salsa still has some texture.

Roasted garlic: Brush garlic cloves with olive oil and put in a small skillet. Cover and cook over medium-low heat, shaking the pan periodically to rotate the garlic, until the cloves are soft inside their skins, 10 to 12 minutes. Remove from the heat and set aside to cool. Pop the garlic cloves out of their skins and use immediately or cover and refrigerate for up to 3 days.

FEELING GREEN: Skip the chipotle and try adding ½ teaspoon of sugar just before pureeing to temper the tomatoes.

FEELING FOOD: Add ½ cup of chopped black olives and serve over Stewed Lentils and Rice (page 136).

FEELING FULL: Serve over grilled fish, chicken, beef, or tofu to get in your veggies.

Creamy Guacamole • MAKES 1½ CUPS

Everyone loves guacamole, and, contrary to what many people think, avocados are good for you: they're filled with heart-healthy fats, as well as vitamin K, fiber, and potassium, a mineral that helps regulate blood pressure. When selecting Hass avocados, choose ripe but firm ones or opt for hard, green avocados and ripen them at home in a paper bag.

1 large Hass avocado
1 tablespoon fresh lime juice
2 teaspoons chopped scallions, white and green parts
1 small jalapeño, seeded and finely chopped
1 tablespoon chopped fresh cilantro
Salt and freshly ground pepper

Halve and pit the avocado and scoop the flesh into a small bowl. Cut it into rough ½-inch chunks with a dinner knife. Add the lime juice, scallions, jalapeño, and cilantro, season with salt and pepper, and mash slightly with a fork. If not using immediately, cover with plastic wrap, pressing it down onto the surface to prevent discoloration, and refrigerate for up to 1 day.

FEELING GREEN: Skip the jalapeño, add a chopped hard-boiled egg, and prepare as directed. Enjoy this protein-fortified spread over whole grain toast or crackers.

FEELING FOOD: Creamy avocado with crunchy tortilla chips—not sure how to improve on that. Maybe a virgin margarita to go with it?

FEELING FULL: This heart-healthy treat will keep you satiated. Make a salad platter of guacamole and your choice of salsa over baby arugula.

Make: Creamy Guacamole (opposite), Salsa Cruda (page 96), and sliced mushrooms and zucchini sautéed in olive oil.

Buy: Soft tortillas, canned black beans, sour cream, shredded cheddar, romaine lettuce, virgin mojito mix, and fresh mint.

To serve: Wrap the tortillas in foil and warm in a 200°F oven. Chop the lettuce and place in a bowl. Put the guacamole, salsa, sour cream, and cheddar in bowls. Heat the black beans and season with salt and pepper. Mash for a smooth but chunky consistency and keep warm. Keep the mushrooms and zucchini warm, too. Bring everything to the table and invite everyone to make her own burrito.

To drink: Divide the mojito mix between two pitchers. Add rum to one of them and differentiate it from the virgin one with fresh mint leaves.

The Picnic Box • SERVES 1

The picnic box is a year-round lunch- or snack-time energy booster. You can keep the ingredients for it in your fridge and, with little effort, whip one up in minutes. It is great for company, yet can, as the name implies, be packed to go: on a plane, to a picnic, on a road trip, or to work. Use your imagination to vary the components as your taste or the season dictates.

1 wedge artisanal cheese of choice
6 olives
Raw vegetables, such as carrots, celery, or cucumber sticks;
    radishes; or whatever is in season
½ cup Classic Hummus (page 92), Tuna Salad (opposite), egg salad,
    or White Bean Dip (page 95)
Whole grain crackers, a slice of good whole grain bread, or a roll

Arrange the ingredients decoratively on a plate or pack them in a portable container. Keep refrigerated until you are ready to go.

FEELING GREEN: Try plain goat cheese, green olives, cucumbers, and the Feeling Green variation of Classic Hummus (page 92) with crackers.

FEELING FOOD: Try Manchego cheese, black olives, carrots, and grape tomatoes with White Bean Dip (page 95) and a roll.

FEELING FULL: Try thinly shaved Parmesan, niçoise olives, and a generous mixture of crudités including turnips, bell pepper strips, and celery sticks. Roll tuna salad in romaine lettuce leaves for a finger food on the go.

Tuna Salad • SERVES 2

It's the details that elevate tuna salad from ho-hum to yum. This recipe was written up in the New York Times *many years ago, when Jen was the executive chef of a gourmet shop in Manhattan. How the individual ingredients are chopped has a real impact on the final product. Tuna is fairly soft, so you want the crunch of pieces of celery and pickles, but raw onion can be overpowering and is best when minced as finely as possible so it flavors the salad subtly.*

  1 (6-ounce) can chunk light tuna in water, well drained
¼ cup chopped celery
  2 tablespoons chopped cornichons or baby gherkin pickles
  1 tablespoon minced red onion
  2 tablespoons mayonnaise
  2 teaspoons minced fresh dill
  Pinch of freshly ground pepper

Mix the tuna, celery, pickles, onion, mayonnaise, dill, and pepper in a small bowl and enjoy! You can keep this for a day or two in the fridge.

FEELING GREEN: Many green-ers who usually cannot do fish still do well with tuna salad. Try it, replacing the onion with minced scallion, or omitting the onion family completely.

FEELING FOOD: This salad works well on toasted whole grain bread, layered with mayonnaise, lettuce, and sliced tomato.

FEELING FULL: Use only 1 table-spoon of mayonnaise when preparing this, or substitute with 1 tablespoon of olive oil and a good squirt of lemon juice. Roll tuna salad inside a large romaine leaf for a light yet filling snack.

ABOUT MERCURY IN TUNA

Since the level of mercury in tuna is a concern, it's useful to know that canned chunk light is the safest (tuna steak has the highest level). The FDA recommends limiting the consumption of tuna to once a week when you are pregnant or nursing. We prefer a more conservative stance of once every three weeks, but the choice is yours. If you are avoiding tuna completely, make this with canned wild Alaskan salmon instead. Be sure to drain the salmon thoroughly and check that it is completely clean of skin and bones.

Bruschetta or Crostini • MAKES 8 SLICES

Bruschetta and crostini are essentially grilled or toasted bread slices, which are seasoned and then served with a variety of toppings. The technical difference between the two is that bruschetta are toasted and then rubbed with garlic, and crostini are brushed with olive oil and then toasted. This recipe combines the best of both methods. Prepare them and call them what you like; they make an exceptional little snack or light lunch. Anything that can be spread or spooned onto a piece of toast is bruschetta/crostini material. See the Feeling . . . variations for topping suggestions.

8 (½-inch-thick) diagonal slices of French baguette,
    or 4 slices of rustic round loaf, halved
1 clove garlic, halved, optional
2 tablespoons extra-virgin olive oil

Preheat a grill pan over medium-high heat or preheat the broiler. Grill the bread slices until well marked and lightly toasted, about 2 minutes per side, or broil on a baking sheet 8 inches away from the heating element until golden, about 2 minutes. Rub the slices of bread with the cut side of the garlic, if using, and then brush with olive oil.

FEELING GREEN: Spread with Tapenade (opposite; though you may want to omit the anchovy option). The salty flavor, accented with fresh lemon juice, could make this snack perfect for you.

FEELING FOOD: Enjoy Goat Cheese with Herbs (page 104). Top with Pesto alla Genovese (page 130) or Sun-Dried Tomato Pesto (page 131) for a mouthwatering treat.

FEELING FULL: Opt for whole grain bread when you make the bruschetta and spoon Classic Bruschetta Topping (page 104) on top.

Tapenade • MAKES 1 CUP

1½ cups pitted black olives, such as niçoise or kalamata
1 small clove garlic, crushed
1 small anchovy, optional
2 teaspoons fresh lemon juice
¼ cup extra-virgin olive oil
  A few grinds of pepper
¼ cup chopped fresh Italian parsley

In the bowl of a food processor, process the olives, garlic, and anchovy to a fairly smooth paste. Add the lemon juice, olive oil, and pepper and process to blend. Add the parsley and pulse several times to incorporate. The tapenade can be kept refrigerated in an airtight container for 2 weeks.

THAT'S ENTERTAINMENT | Viva Italia!

Make: Plain and/or seasoned Bruschetta or Crostini (page 102) and your choice of Classic Bruschetta Topping (page 104), Tapenade (above), Pesto alla Genovese (page 130), Sun-Dried Tomato Pesto (page 131), and/or Goat Cheese with Herbs (page 104).

Buy: Italian cheese, such as bocconcini (small balls of fresh mozzarella) and chunks of Parmesan, fresh baguette, breadsticks, roasted red peppers, artichoke hearts, fresh rosemary, and pomegranate juice.

To serve: Create a platter. Put the bruschetta toppings, roasted peppers, and artichoke hearts in separate bowls. Shave thin Parmesan slices and place in between the bowls. Arrange the bruschetta on a plate. On a separate platter, place a bowl of bocconcini near a bowl of olive oil with a sprig of rosemary in it. Cut up a fresh baguette and arrange around the bowls. Stand the breadsticks in a glass.

To drink: Wine, of course, as well as some pomegranate juice in a carafe for you.

Goat Cheese with Herbs • MAKES ABOUT 1 CUP

1 (6-ounce) log fresh goat cheese
2 tablespoons chopped fresh herbs, such as chives, basil, tarragon,
    and/or dill; or a mixture of 1 teaspoon dried thyme, 1 teaspoon dried
    rosemary, and 2 teaspoons chopped fresh chives
  Freshly ground pepper

Let the goat cheese sit at room temperature for 15 minutes to soften. In a small bowl, mix the cheese with the herbs and pepper until well blended. Use immediately or keep refrigerated for up to 5 days.

Classic Bruschetta Topping • MAKES 1 CUP

3 very red medium plum tomatoes, seeded and chopped
1 tablespoon sliced fresh basil
1 tablespoon extra-virgin olive oil
  Salt and freshly ground pepper

Combine the tomatoes, basil, and olive oil in a bowl and season with salt and pepper.

REAL WORLD

Now that I'm seven months into my pregnancy, I find I don't usually have the energy to prepare a fresh, homemade snack, so what I loved about the bruschetta and tomato topping is that it took less than 10 minutes from start to finish, and the result was well worth it. Fresh basil was definitely key here, and I opted for cut-up cherry tomatoes, my favorite. The garlic was great because it contributed a little bite, and I was liberal with the salt to satisfy that craving. I was pretty casual with the baguette slicing and ended up with pieces of irregular thicknesses. All were good, though I have to admit the ½-inch-thick pieces, as recommended, were definitely the best. They came out crispy and held their crunch when I spooned on the juicy tomato topping. The result was the perfect mix of warm and cold, crunchy and soft. Delicious! Next time I might invest an additional few minutes and try out the goat cheese as well—but for now I was thrilled with the discovery of a craving-worthy new snack and a great, easy appetizer.

Sylvie Tendler, Montreal, Canada

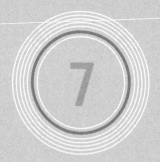

7

⠿ Entrees

In a show on new mothers, Oprah was asking fathers about their perspective on having a new baby at home. One father noted that prior to having the baby, every night when he came home, his wife would greet him at the door with a big smile and a hug. Since she had the baby, though, she looked tired and depleted, meaning no smile, no hug, and no greeting at the door. He said that all he wanted was for her to do that now, to which his wife replied:

"You want a hug when you come home?"

"Yeah."

"Then bring dinner."

Certainly, when your energy is low and you are at your hungriest, dinner is the hardest meal to plan and prepare. Add to that a newborn or some toddlers, and that pizza delivery guy becomes hard to resist. But before you call, check out some of the easy-to-assemble and quick-to-cook recipes that follow. There are chicken and beef dishes that cook up in a single skillet and yield great taste for minimal effort. Several fish dishes can be ready in twenty minutes or less, and there are some fast pastas and a killer stir-fry. And when you have a few extra minutes, the marinated dishes and a slow-cooking chili will surely reward the time you invest.

So grab a handful of nuts or some other snack, put down the phone, and try out a quick and healthy dinner that you will not regret in the morning. Or, greet your spouse at the door with a big hug and this book—turned to whatever you'd like to request for dinner.

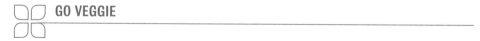

GO VEGGIE

As a longtime vegetarian who feeds a family of carnivores, I know firsthand just how frustrating dinnertime can be for the cook trying to nourish and please everyone. Look for "Go Veggie" boxes throughout for you or the vegetarian in your life.

Broiled Salmon with Caramelized Fennel and Sweet Onion • SERVES 4

This oft-requested Mothers & Menus dish has our moms digging into their omega-3s. If you have never had caramelized fennel before, you are in for a treat. The process softens and sweetens the fennel, while retaining its anise flavor, resulting in a topping that complements salmon's rich texture and works well with other fish, too. Caramelizing is a cooking technique that takes a little practice, so if your vegetables look more sautéed than caramelized, do not despair! They will still be delicious. When Rachel (see Real World, opposite) was pregnant with Avra, this salmon dish was one of her favorites. In her seventh month of pregnancy with a second child, Rachel was feeling nauseated and avoided fish as much as possible, but this tried-and-true recipe got her back in the kitchen.

1 medium sweet onion

1 medium bulb fennel

2 tablespoons olive oil

½ to 1 cup dry white wine; or chicken or vegetable stock, homemade (page 66 or 67) or store-bought, or water

Salt and freshly ground pepper

4 (5- to 6-ounce) skinless wild salmon fillets, about 1 inch thick

1 medium shallot, sliced

1 tablespoon chopped fresh dill, or ½ teaspoon dried

Lemon wedges for garnish

Cut the onion in half and cut each half into ¼-inch-thick slices. Do the same with the fennel.

Heat 1 tablespoon of the oil in a large skillet over medium-low heat. Add the fennel and onion and cook until thoroughly tender, stirring occasionally, about 25 minutes.

Preheat the broiler.

Increase the heat to medium-high under the fennel and onion and cook for about 10 minutes more, stirring occasionally, until the vegetables brown nicely. If a brown residue builds up in the pan, add up to ½ cup of wine and scrape the pan to incorporate any bits back into the vegetable mixture. Season with salt and pepper and keep warm.

Meanwhile, prepare the salmon. Use 1 teaspoon of oil to grease a baking dish. Season the fillets with salt and pepper and put them in the dish. Pour ½ cup of the wine into the dish and scatter the shallot in the wine. Sprinkle with half of the dill and drizzle with the remaining 2 teaspoons of olive oil. Broil the salmon 6 inches away from the heating element for 9 to 12 minutes for medium, until the fish is firm and golden brown, and it flakes when poked with a fork.

To serve, place each fillet on a plate. Spoon a bit of the pan juices over the fish and top with a heaping tablespoon of caramelized vegetables. Garnish each serving with a sprinkling of the remaining dill and add a lemon wedge.

FEELING GREEN: If you can still handle the thought of fish, this recipe may work well for you. If you try it with a milder fish, such as tilapia, reduce the broiling time to 6 to 9 minutes.

FEELING FOOD: The sweet and creamy flavors of this dish work well with Orzo with Spinach, Lemon, Olive Oil, and Herbs (page 166).

FEELING FULL: Enjoy this delicious dish with Balsamic-Glazed Beets (page 146) and a salad with Orange Vinaigrette (page 71) to complement the flavors.

REAL WORLD

Wow, wow, wow. This recipe is amazing. Definitely the best fish I have had since being pregnant and something I look forward to preparing afterwards. I eliminated the dill, not being a fan of it. The shallots on top of the salmon were a great touch and added a lot of flavor. I was pleasantly full after the meal, which rarely happens. I should add that my husband, Richard, is the real cook in the family and my forays into the kitchen have often turned out badly (though well meaning). But this dish turned out superbly and Richard and I both really enjoyed it.

Rachel, Brooklyn, NY

GO VEGGIE

Elevate Seared Tofu (see page 138) with a topping of caramelized fennel for a delicious entree.

Broiled Halibut Provençal • SERVES 4

Seasoned with fresh herbs and flavored with white wine and Slow-Roasted Tomatoes (page 133), this simple and tasty entree draws rave reviews from health-conscious moms. (Time-conscious moms should check out the Express tip, below.)

2 tablespoons olive oil, plus extra for the baking dish
1 tablespoon finely chopped fresh herbs, such as rosemary, thyme, chives, or sweet marjoram, or a combination
1 clove garlic, minced
1 medium shallot, minced
½ cup dry white wine or vegetable stock, homemade (page 67) or store-bought
4 (6-ounce) skinless halibut fillets, about 1 inch thick
Salt and freshly ground pepper
1 cup chopped Slow-Roasted Tomatoes (page 133)
Chopped fresh Italian parsley for garnish
Lemon wedges for garnish

Preheat the broiler. Lightly oil a 10 × 13-inch baking dish.

In a medium bowl, mix together the herbs, garlic, shallot, wine, and the 2 tablespoons of olive oil. Dip the fillets into the herb mixture, coating well on both sides. Place the fish in the baking dish and pour the remaining herb mixture over the fillets. Season with salt and pepper.

Broil for 6 minutes about 3 inches from the heating element.

Scatter the chopped tomatoes over the fish, spoon the pan juices on top of the tomatoes, and continue broiling until the fillets flake when poked with a fork, 2 to 4 minutes. Serve immediately, garnished with parsley and lemon wedges.

Express: Replace the Slow-Roasted Tomatoes with 4 medium plum tomatoes, seeded and chopped. Toss with the herbs, garlic, shallot, wine, and olive oil, and spoon on top of the fish. Broil for 8 to 10 minutes, until the fish is cooked.

FEELING GREEN: If you are doing well with fish, then this dish might work for you, especially when accompanied by Potato and Celery Root Puree (page 171).

FEELING FOOD: Enjoy this dish, prepared as indicated, with *gratin dauphinois* (the Feeling Food version of Creamless Potato Gratin on page 172).

FEELING FULL: Turn this dish into a tuna-free and mercury-safe take on *salade niçoise* by adding greens, olives, steamed green beans, and a hard-boiled egg (skip the boiled potato). Dress with Lemon-Dijon Vinaigrette (page 77) or Sherry Vinaigrette (page 73).

Tilapia Veracruzana • SERVES 4

When Jen's daughter, Jyah, graduated from high school, they took a mother-daughter journey to the Yucatán Peninsula in Mexico. Around four o'clock every afternoon, local fishermen would pull their rowboats onto the beach and offer up the day's catch. That night, the fish would be written up on a chalkboard of the local restaurant as the catch of the day and offered with a choice of sauces. Their favorite was the salsa Veracruzana, a richly flavored, lemon-scented blend of tomatoes, green olives, capers, and thyme with a slight kick of jalapeño. Now our mothers enjoy this delicious sauce on tilapia or whatever wild fish looks good at the market.

2 tablespoons olive oil, plus additional to rub on the tilapia

1 small yellow onion, thinly sliced

2 cloves garlic, minced

1 jalapeño, seeded and chopped

4 ripe red tomatoes (about 1 pound), seeded and cut into ½-inch chunks

1 bay leaf

1 teaspoon grated lemon zest

1 tablespoon chopped fresh thyme

½ cup sliced pitted green olives, either manzanilla or cerignola

2 tablespoons drained capers

Salt and freshly ground pepper

4 (5- to 6-ounce) tilapia fillets, about 1 inch thick

1 lemon, cut into wedges

Heat the oil in a skillet over medium heat. Add the onion, garlic, and jalapeño and cook, stirring frequently, until softened, about 5 minutes. Raise the heat to medium-high and add the tomatoes, bay leaf, lemon zest, thyme, olives, and capers. Cook until some of the liquid evaporates, about 5 minutes. Reduce the heat and cook for 10 minutes more to let the flavors meld. Season to taste with salt and pepper and cool. The sauce can be made in advance and refrigerated overnight. Bring to room temperature before serving.

Preheat the broiler.

Rub the tilapia fillets with a little olive oil, spritz with lemon juice, and season with salt and pepper. Place in a shallow baking dish and broil, about 3 inches from the heating element until the fish flakes when poked with a fork, 8 to 10 minutes.

Place the tilapia on plates, spoon the sauce over it, garnish with a lemon wedge, and serve immediately.

FEELING GREEN: The combination of flavors in this dish is beautiful for when you are feeling good, but it is not a good match for a queasy stomach. Instead, try the Broiled Halibut Provençal (page 110) with a side of Orzo with Spinach, Lemon, Olive Oil, and Herbs (page 166).

FEELING FOOD: Use your favorite fish for this dish and accompany with Herb-Roasted Potatoes (page 168) and Sautéed Zucchini and Yellow Squash with Baby Tomatoes and Dill (page 154).

FEELING FULL: This delicious fish dish may become your summer staple! Accompany with Corn Salad on Baby Greens with Avocado and Feta (page 87) or Sugar Snap Peas with Tomato and Mint (page 145) to round this out into a full meal.

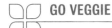 **GO VEGGIE**

This is a great dish to prepare for a mixed group of vegetarians and fish eaters. Prepare the salsa as directed and then broil some fish as directed and pan-sear tofu (see page 138). You can also sear some chicken breasts to give everyone a taste of her favorite entree.

Miso-Glazed Salmon • SERVES 4

Coupling miso paste with wild salmon makes this a powerful, heart-healthy, craveable entree that is also quick and easy to prepare. You can continue the Asian theme by serving it with Asian Cabbage Salad (page 80) or Seaweed Salad (page 82) and Sesame Lotus Root Soba Noodles (page 167). Or keep it simple and pair the salmon with steamed brown rice (see page 173) and salad greens dressed with Carrot-Ginger Dressing (page 83).

¼ cup red or white miso paste
2 tablespoons fresh orange juice
1 tablespoon toasted sesame oil
1 tablespoon honey
1 tablespoon peeled and grated fresh ginger
Pinch of cayenne pepper
4 (5- to 6-ounce) wild salmon fillets, about 1 inch thick
Black sesame seeds for garnish, optional
Lemon or lime wedges for garnish

Preheat the broiler.

To make the glaze, stir together the miso, juice, oil, honey, ginger, and cayenne in a small bowl.

Put the salmon fillets in a shallow baking dish and pour the glaze over them. Broil about 3 inches from the heating element, spooning the glaze over the fillets twice during cooking, until firm and golden brown, a total of 12 minutes for medium.

To serve, place the fillets on plates, top with any remaining glaze, and sprinkle with sesame seeds. Serve immediately with lemon or lime wedges.

FEELING GREEN: The salty, tangy flavor of the miso paste may be appealing. If you find the flavor of salmon to be too robust, try a milder white fish. Accompany with a simple grain of your choice and a roasted vegetable, such as asparagus (see page 155).

FEELING FOOD: Enjoy this dish, prepared as indicated, with Crisp Roasted Sweet Potatoes (page 169) and Green Beans with Carrots, Shallots, and Thyme (page 150).

FEELING FULL: The only way to improve on this epitome of a healthy, satisfying dish would be to pair it with your favorite sautéed greens (see page 152) and ½ cup steamed quinoa (see page 173).

REAL WORLD

As a Jewish Italian, most of my recipes are very familiar, and I never have ingredients like miso paste or sesame oil in my home. But I love eating at Asian restaurants, so I thought this would be a great opportunity to try cooking this kind of food at home. I could not believe how easy it was, how fast it was, and how delicious it was. The finished dish tasted a lot like the miso cod at Nobu's, which I love! Every time I eat there I am amazed at how intricate the tastes are, and here I was making it at home, in no time! The glaze seems so versatile to me; I am going to try it out on other fish too, starting with cod. The only change I made was omitting the ginger from the glaze, because I just don't like it. Noah, twelve months, surprised me by eating the fish and asking for more. He is a great eater, but I hadn't expected him to enjoy the Asian flavorings. And my husband, Steven, was just thrilled at the change in the dinner menu. I wanted to make some side dishes, too, so I tried out the Sesame Lotus Root Soba Noodles (excellent!) and the Sugar Snap Peas with Tomato and Mint (Yum!). As a dentist who truly believes that you are what you eat, I was pleased to find easy and delicious options for making such healthy foods.

Melanie Englese, New York, NY

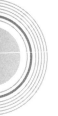

Sautéed Chicken Cutlets with Sun-Dried Tomatoes and Herbs • SERVES 4

This one-pan, crowd-pleasing dish comes together in less than 15 minutes. You want to use cutlets that are thin enough to cook through on the stovetop. You can slice (or have your butcher slice) the chicken breasts horizontally, or you can cut them into pieces and then pound them (which can be a great stress-relieving activity!). Or you can buy thin cutlets that are all ready to go.

½ cup sliced sun-dried tomatoes

1 tablespoon minced fresh rosemary

¼ cup fresh lemon juice

¼ cup chicken stock, homemade (page 66) or store-bought

8 (3-ounce) chicken breast cutlets

Salt and freshly ground pepper

¼ cup olive oil

2 cloves garlic, minced

¼ cup white wine, or additional stock

1 tablespoon chopped fresh Italian parsley

If the tomatoes are dry-packed, put them in a bowl, add hot water to cover, and let soak for 5 minutes. Drain and return to the bowl. (If they are packed in oil, simply drain.) Toss with the rosemary, lemon juice, and stock. Set aside.

Rinse the cutlets and pat dry. Season with salt and pepper.

Heat the olive oil in a large, heavy skillet over medium-high heat. Add the chicken and cook until golden brown, about 2 minutes on each side. Add the garlic, cook for 1 minute, and then add the wine. Cook for 1 minute before adding the tomatoes and the parsley. Cook until the chicken is cooked through and the sauce is slightly reduced, 3 to 4 minutes. Serve immediately.

FEELING GREEN: Prepare sautéed chicken cutlets with lemon and herbs instead. Omit the sun-dried tomatoes and follow the recipe as directed, adding 1 tablespoon of chopped fresh dill or tarragon. Enjoy with a side of steamed grains, such as millet, rice, or quinoa (see page 173), and your favorite roasted vegetable.

FEELING FOOD: Try Marie's variation (see Real World, below) for a richer, deeper taste that cooking skin-on, bone-in dark meat provides. Accompany with the Feeling Food variations of Crisp Roasted Sweet Potatoes (page 169) and some mixed greens with Balsamic Vinaigrette (page 73).

FEELING FULL: Take this dish out of the pan and into the broiler for a highly flavorful variation that uses less olive oil and salt. Preheat the broiler. Omit the sun-dried tomatoes, and reduce the olive oil to 1 tablespoon. Toss the chicken with rosemary, lemon juice, stock, oil, garlic, and salt and pepper. Broil the chicken until golden brown, turning once, about 4 to 5 minutes on each side. Serve immediately with pan juices.

REAL WORLD

Our family prefers chicken with the skin on, so I tried the recipe out using whole chicken legs—delicious! The result was very tasty and nourishing with a deep, rich flavor that we all enjoyed. I was actually surprised that our fifteen-month-old son, Asker, enjoyed the sun-dried tomatoes; that was nice. Because I used bone-in legs, I did increase the cooking time. I also used only 2 tablespoons of olive oil because the skin gave off some fat and juices. I cooked them on each side for 4 to 5 minutes, and then added some chicken stock and let them simmer, covered, for about 12 minutes more. Then I continued the recipe as directed, adding some chopped onion (which we love) along with the garlic. The finished dish was really yummy.

Marie Lumholtz, Olivebridge, NY

Grilled Chicken with Summer Salsa • SERVES 4

This makes a great entree for the dog days of summer, perfect for outdoor cooking but certainly adaptable to the broiler. Tomato, fresh corn, and avocado combine to complement the lime-and-cumin–scented chicken. Add a big green salad and roasted baby potatoes, and you've got a splendid meal.

The chicken needs to marinate for at least 3 hours, so consider preparing it in the morning, along with the salsa base, so that you can pull together a quick lunch or dinner.

Grated zest and juice of 1 large lime
2 tablespoons olive oil
4 cloves garlic, minced
1 teaspoon ground cumin
$\frac{1}{2}$ teaspoon freshly ground pepper
1 (3$\frac{1}{2}$-pound) chicken, cut in 8 pieces;
    or 4 bone-in, skin-on chicken breast halves
Coarse salt
Summer Salsa (recipe follows)

In a glass or another nonreactive baking dish, combine the zest, lime juice, olive oil, garlic, cumin, and pepper. Add the chicken, coat thoroughly with the marinade, and refrigerate for at least 3 hours or overnight, turning once.

Prepare a medium-hot fire in a charcoal grill, preheat a gas grill to medium-high, or preheat the broiler.

Season the chicken with salt and grill until cooked through, about 8 minutes per side for breasts and 12 minutes per side for dark meat. Place the chicken on plates and spoon the salsa alongside.

Summer Salsa • MAKES 2 CUPS

Fresh corn, juicy tomatoes, and fragrant cilantro combine great color and taste in a summer side that perks up any dish.

1 cup fresh corn kernels (2 ears)
1 large beefsteak tomato, seeded and diced
1 small jalapeño, seeded and minced
1 scallion, white and green parts, chopped fine
½ cup chopped fresh cilantro
1 tablespoon extra-virgin olive oil
1 teaspoon fresh lime juice
1 medium avocado, preferably Hass
Salt and freshly ground pepper

Bring 1 or 2 inches of water to a boil in the bottom of a steamer or in a medium pot fitted with a steamer insert. Add the corn, cover the steamer, and steam until the corn is tender, about 5 minutes. Drain the corn.

Combine the corn, tomato, jalapeño, scallion, cilantro, olive oil, and ½ teaspoon of the lime juice. (This can be done up to 6 hours in advance; refrigerate the salsa.) To serve, pit, peel, and chop the avocado into ½-inch chunks. Toss with the remaining ½ teaspoon of lime juice, add the avocado to the salsa, and season to taste with salt and pepper.

FEELING GREEN: With its fresh and light flavors, this dish may serve you well. Omit the cumin in the marinade and omit the jalapeño from the salsa.

FEELING FOOD: Prepare the Summer Salsa as directed, but omit the avocado. Use it to make Creamy Guacamole (page 98) instead, and enjoy the two side by side with the chicken.

FEELING FULL: Enjoy this delicious entree without altering the recipe and pair it with the Summer Vegetable Salad (page 85) for a delicious, nutrient-packed meal.

Balsamic and Herb-Roasted Chicken • SERVES 4

This is not your run-of-the-mill roast chicken. The caramelized vinegar creates a sweet and crisp skin, which is complemented by fragrant herbs. The result is robust, juicy, and downright delicious!

2 branches fresh rosemary

1 (3½-pound) chicken

2 sprigs fresh marjoram, optional

1 medium sweet onion, quartered

2 cloves garlic, peeled

½ cup good-quality balsamic vinegar

2 tablespoons fresh lemon juice

½ cup chicken stock, homemade (page 66) or store-bought

1 tablespoon olive oil

Coarse sea or kosher salt and freshly ground pepper

Preheat the oven to 400°F.

Finely chop enough of the rosemary leaves to make 2 tablespoons. Set aside. Cut the branches into 1-inch pieces.

Remove the giblets and any excess fat from the chicken. Rinse the bird thoroughly and pat dry. Loosen the skin around the breast and thigh by gently running your index finger or thumb under the skin. Tuck the pieces of rosemary branch under the skin, along the thigh and breast.

Lay the chicken breast side up in a roasting pan. Put the marjoram, onion, and garlic inside the cavity of the chicken.

Whisk together the vinegar, lemon juice, and stock and pour over the chicken. Rub with the olive oil and sprinkle with 1 tablespoon of the chopped rosemary and salt and pepper.

Turn the chicken breast side down. Season the underside of the chicken with the remaining tablespoon of chopped rosemary and more salt and pepper.

Transfer the pan to the oven and roast the chicken for 30 minutes. Turn the chicken breast side up and baste with pan juices. Roast, basting frequently, until the skin is a deep golden brown and the thigh juices run clear when pierced with the tip of a small sharp knife, 45 to 50 minutes.

Remove the chicken to a platter or cutting board and allow it to rest for 10 minutes before carving. Skim and discard the fat from the pan juices and serve the pan juices alongside the chicken.

FEELING GREEN: Do not attempt this in your state! Instead, put 4 (8-ounce) bone-in, skin-on chicken breast halves in a roasting pan. Whisk together the vinegar, lemon juice, stock, and olive oil and pour over the breasts. Place rosemary branches (with the leaves on) in the pan under the chicken. Omit the chopped rosemary, marjoram, onion, and garlic. Roast for 30 minutes. Remove the herb branches prior to serving. Pair with the Herb-Roasted Potatoes (page 168) and Green Beans with Carrots, Shallots, and Thyme (page 150).

FEELING FOOD: For a soothing, balanced, meal, pair this roasted chicken with the Feeling Food variations of Potato and Celery Root Puree (page 171) and some Asian-Style Roasted Broccoli (page 156) or Roasted Cauliflower with Curry (page 157).

FEELING FULL: Enjoy, enjoy, enjoy. Add the Spinach, Pine Nuts, and Golden Raisins (page 144) and some Crisp Roasted Sweet Potatoes (page 169) for a beautifully balanced meal.

Seared Beef Tenderloin with Port and Mushrooms • SERVES 2

This Mothers & Menus favorite is a great source of iron, which is essential during pregnancy. And the port sauce is sexy and delicious, which are essential qualities any time.

> 2 (6-ounce) beef tenderloin steaks, 1½ inches thick
> Coarse salt and freshly ground pepper
> 2 tablespoons olive oil
> 1 medium shallot, minced
> 8 ounces mushrooms, preferably shiitake and cremini, trimmed and sliced
> 1 teaspoon chopped fresh rosemary
> ½ cup ruby port, or additional stock
> ½ cup chicken stock, homemade (page 66) or store-bought

Season the beef on both sides with salt and pepper, and brush with 1 tablespoon of the olive oil.

Heat a heavy skillet over medium-high heat until very hot. Brown the steaks for 4 minutes on each side for medium-rare and remove to a plate.

Add the remaining 1 tablespoon of olive oil to the pan along with the shallot and sauté for 1 minute. Add the mushrooms and sauté until the mushrooms are a deep brown and any moisture has evaporated, 6 to 8 minutes. Add the rosemary and port and simmer, scraping up any browned bits on the bottom of the pan, until the liquid has reduced and is almost syrupy, 2 to 3 minutes. Add the stock and reduce over medium-heat until almost syrupy, 2 to 3 minutes.

Spoon the port sauce over the steaks and serve immediately.

FEELING GREEN: Increasing iron intake is said to alleviate morning sickness. The shallot balances out the sweetness of the wine, but if your nausea is aggravated by anything in the onion family, just skip it.

FEELING FOOD: Pair this dish with Herb-Roasted Potatoes (page 168) and creamed spinach (see the Feeling Food variation on page 144) for a healthy take on *steak frites* (steak and fries).

FEELING FULL: Try this with the Spinach, Pine Nuts, and Golden Raisins (page 144) and a simple salad of baby greens with your favorite dressing to help with digestion.

ABOUT COOKING WITH WINE

Cooking with wine is a great way to enjoy its sophisticated taste without indulging. But alcohol's evaporation depends on the amount of time it spends on the stovetop. While dishes that have simmered for hours have been shown to have little of the added alcohol left in them (about 5 percent), dishes that are cooked more quickly can retain anywhere from 10 to 50 percent. Now, if you are using only ½ cup of wine to make a pan sauce for four, for example, even if the wine retains half of its initial alcohol once cooked, you would be consuming the equivalent of 1 tablespoon of wine with your portion. If you want to avoid alcohol completely, simply use the nonalcoholic option provided with each recipe.

GO VEGGIE

This mushroom and wine sauce works great served alongside Seared Tofu (see page 138). Just follow the directions for the sauce preparation and serve with the tofu. If you are having vegetarian guests for dinner, this works out perfectly—just make sure to use a different pan when preparing the sauce from the one you used to cook the meat.

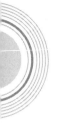

Baked Fusilli with Classic Marinara Sauce, Ricotta, and Parmesan • SERVES 4

This mild-flavored sweet sauce, enhanced by the lightness of ricotta and just the right amount of Parmesan, results in a creamy pasta dish that is absolutely delicious, without being heavy. Try it with Sautéed Kale (page 147), Sautéed Bitter Greens with Shallots (page 152), or Mama's Turkey Meatballs (page 126).

8 ounces dried fusilli, penne, or another pasta shape

1 tablespoon extra-virgin olive oil, plus extra for the baking dish

2 tablespoons chopped fresh Italian parsley

2 cups Classic Marinara Sauce (recipe follows)

Salt and freshly ground pepper

1 cup ricotta

½ cup freshly grated Parmesan cheese

Preheat the oven to 375°F.

Cook the pasta according to the package directions. Drain and toss with the olive oil, parsley, and 1 cup of the marinara.

Lightly oil an 8 × 8-inch baking dish. Put the pasta in the dish and spoon the remaining cup of marinara on top, smoothing it with the back of the spoon. Cover the pasta with dollops of ricotta and sprinkle with the Parmesan. Loosely cover the dish with foil and bake until the cheeses are melted, about 20 minutes.

In a pinch: Replace Classic Marinara Sauce with your favorite jarred marinara sauce; use shredded mozzarella in place of Parmesan. If you have no ricotta, just skip it, and add additional Parmesan or mozzarella instead.

FEELING GREEN: When you are feeling green, a thick, tomato-filled sauce may make you even more uncomfortable. Replace the marinara sauce with Slow-Roasted Tomatoes (page 133). Sneak in some greens by finely chopping spinach or kale and stirring into the ricotta.

FEELING FOOD: Add 2 tablespoons of heavy cream to the finished sauce. Enjoy with some Bruschetta or Crostini (page 102) and a green salad.

FEELING FULL: Use whole grain pasta such as quinoa rotelle by the Quinoa Corporation. Undercook it slightly when boiling, as quinoa pasta can go from yum to mush quickly. You can also use whole wheat pasta; spoon ½ cup of additional sauce over the top before baking.

Classic Marinara Sauce • MAKES 2 QUARTS

This naturally sweet tomato sauce freezes beautifully, and is great to have around for last-minute dinners. To pump up the nutrients in the marinara, add 1 medium zucchini or yellow squash, finely diced, in the last 15 minutes of the simmer.

¼ cup olive oil

1 medium sweet onion, chopped

3 cloves garlic, minced

1 medium carrot, finely chopped

1 bay leaf

2 (28-ounce) cans whole plum tomatoes, with their juice

2 tablespoons chopped fresh oregano, or 1 teaspoon dried

¼ cup chopped fresh basil, or 1½ tablespoons dried

Salt and freshly ground pepper

Heat the oil in a large, heavy saucepan over medium heat. Add the onion, garlic, carrot, and bay leaf and cook, stirring occasionally, until softened, about 5 minutes.

Add the tomatoes and reduce the heat to low. Simmer, partially covered, until slightly reduced, 30 minutes. Add the oregano and basil and cook for another 5 minutes. Remove from the heat.

With an immersion blender, pulse the sauce several times until it is pureed but still has some texture. Alternatively, use a regular blender. Season to taste with salt and pepper.

Mama's Turkey Meatballs • SERVES 4

Jen's mama, Carla, is Sicilian and knows a thing or two about meatballs. Jen updated this favorite classic with turkey to create a healthy alternative to traditional meatballs, made with beef. Serve these with Classic Marinara Sauce (page 125) over whole wheat spaghetti. If you have any leftovers, make a healthy hero sandwich by spooning some sauce onto a whole grain roll, placing some meatballs on top, sprinkling with Parmesan, and broiling in the toaster oven.

This mixture works well shaped into a hamburger, and broiled or grilled. Double up on the recipe to freeze for later use: Shape the mixture into meatballs or patties, lay out on a sheet of aluminum foil, wrap well, and freeze. Defrost overnight in the fridge before cooking.

> 1 pound ground turkey
> ¼ cup minced yellow onion
> 1 clove garlic, minced
> 1 tablespoon chopped fresh Italian parsley
> 1 tablespoon chopped fresh thyme
> ½ teaspoon cayenne pepper, optional
> ½ cup plain dry bread crumbs
> 1 large egg
> 1 teaspoon salt
> ½ teaspoon freshly ground pepper
> 2 tablespoons olive oil

In a medium bowl, with your hands, combine the turkey, onion, garlic, parsley, thyme, cayenne, bread crumbs, egg, salt, and pepper. Shape into 2-inch meatballs.

In a large skillet, heat the olive oil over medium-high heat. Add the meatballs and brown on all sides, about 5 minutes. Reduce the heat, cover the pan, and cook until cooked through, about 15 minutes.

FEELING GREEN: Omit the onion, cayenne, and bread crumbs. Add ½ cup (uncooked) plain white rice to the meat mixture before shaping. In a medium pot, bring 1 quart of chicken stock, homemade (page 66) or store-bought, to a boil. Drop the meatballs in gently, return the soup to a boil, and reduce the heat so that it simmers. Cover and cook until the meatballs are cooked through, 20 to 25 minutes. Enjoy as a soothing soup or remove meatballs from the soup and enjoy over a bowl of pasta or rice.

FEELING FOOD: Add ¼ cup of grated Parmesan to the mixture and prepare as directed.

FEELING FULL: Look for ground turkey breast, which naturally contains less fat than dark meat. Replace the bread crumbs with ½ cup of cooked millet (see page 173). Preheat the oven to 450°F. Line a baking sheet with aluminum foil and drizzle with olive oil. Put the meatballs on the sheet and drizzle with olive oil. Bake until the meatballs are cooked through, 15 to 20 minutes.

GO VEGGIE

This recipe works great with ground soy protein (make sure to look for non-GMO, such as Smart Ground by Lightlife). Replace the turkey meat with 1 pound of ground soy protein for delicious results. Keep in mind that soy protein is a processed food, and should be treated as one in terms of its frequency in your diet. But when you are craving spaghetti and meatballs or a burger, this will do the trick!

REAL WORLD

I used the Feeling Full suggestion of baking the meatballs instead of panfrying them. They are excellent. I use an ice-cream scoop instead of my hands to shape the meatballs—I came up with that idea when my kids were young and wanted to help out in the kitchen. We also made the Baked Fusilli with Marinara Sauce, Ricotta, and Parmesan [page 124]. It was so easy to make. It's usually hard to impress this pasta-loving family, but these dishes were just delicious. I can't wait to try the fettuccine and mushroom dish!

Charli Bohm, Ocean, NJ

Best Turkey Bolognese · SERVES 6 TO 8

Traditionally, Bolognese is made with a mixture of beef, pork, and veal, which yields a rich, delicious, but not-so-healthy sauce. This recipe yields yummy results without compromising on nutritional value.

  3 tablespoons olive oil
  1 medium sweet onion, diced
  1 medium carrot, peeled and diced
  1 stalk celery, finely diced
  3 cloves garlic, minced
1½ pounds ground turkey
  1 cup dry red or white wine, or chicken or vegetable stock,
    homemade (page 66 or 67) or store-bought
¼ cup tomato paste
  1 (28-ounce) can whole plum tomatoes, with their juice
  1 bay leaf
  1 teaspoon salt
  1 tablespoon chopped fresh oregano, or 1 teaspoon dried
  2 teaspoons chopped fresh thyme, ½ teaspoon dried
    Freshly ground pepper
  1 (16-ounce) box spaghetti

In a large saucepan, heat the olive oil over medium heat and add the onion, carrot, celery, and garlic. Cook the vegetables, stirring frequently, until the onions are translucent but not brown, about 5 minutes. Add the ground turkey and cook until brown, about 10 minutes. Increase the heat to medium-high, add the wine, and cook until the wine is almost completely evaporated, about 5 minutes. Add the tomato paste, tomatoes and their juice, bay leaf, and the salt. Crush the tomatoes with the back of a wooden spoon. Reduce the heat and simmer, uncovered, stirring occasionally, for 1 hour. Add the oregano and thyme and continue simmering until the sauce is thick, about 30 minutes. Adjust the seasoning with additional salt and some pepper.

When the sauce is nearly done, cook the pasta according to the package directions. Drain well, transfer to bowls, and top with the sauce.

FEELING GREEN: When adding the tomatoes and their juice, add a teaspoon of sugar to the sauce. This old folk remedy has not yet been substantiated by research, but seems to be helpful to many who suffer from the acidity in tomatoes.

FEELING FOOD: This classic comfort dish is best accompanied by freshly grated Parmigiano-Reggiano.

FEELING FULL: Double the carrot and celery and prepare as directed. Instead of cooking spaghetti, ladle the sauce over a bowl of cooked quinoa or millet (see page 173). You may also want to explore pasta made from quinoa or another whole grain for a more pasta-like meal. While these are relatively processed, they make a great alternative to traditional semolina flour.

REAL WORLD

This recipe was so easy and quick, I loved it. I am not good with improvising in the kitchen, so I basically stuck to the recipe. The only change I made was to add in an additional carrot and celery because I like more vegetables in my sauce. My husband, Itay, makes Bolognese sauce all the time with veal, beef, milk, and lots of wine. So he was very surprised at how good this tastes and also at how much easier it was! I was happy with how much lighter it felt. We tried it over elbow pasta so I could get the girls, Zoe, four, and Emma, twenty months, to taste it, and found it to be surprisingly good (we usually go with spaghetti).

Lilly Berelovich, Radburn, NJ

Linguine with Pesto alla Genovese • SERVES 6 TO 8

You can buy beautiful basil year-round to make this sauce, a heady and healthful addition to pasta, grilled chicken, fish, or vegetables. You can double up on this classic pesto recipe from Genoa and keep half in the refrigerator to use as a delicious topping for Bruschetta or Crostini (page 102) or as a delightful salad dressing (see the Feeling Green variation, opposite). Pesto will keep in the refrigerator for up to 1 week, or in the freezer for 1 month. Seal the surface of the pesto with a thin layer of oil to prevent discoloration.

1 (16-ounce) box linguine or another long pasta, such as fettucine or spaghetti
1 cup freshly grated Parmesan cheese
$^2/_3$ cup pine nuts
2 cloves garlic, peeled
$^1/_2$ to $^3/_4$ cup extra-virgin olive oil
4 cups loosely packed basil leaves
Salt and freshly ground pepper

Cook the pasta according to the package directions.

While the pasta is cooking, in the bowl of a food processor, grind the cheese, pine nuts, and garlic with $^1/_2$ cup of the olive oil until a smooth paste forms. Add the basil and puree until smooth, adding more oil as needed to make a thick, but not dry, paste. Add salt and pepper to taste.

Drain the pasta and toss with the pesto sauce.

Express: For a delicious picnic lunch or summer dinner, cook a pound of whole grain pasta shapes, toss with pesto—homemade or store-bought—and add any or all of the following (chill for whatever time you have):

- Halved grape or cherry tomatoes
- Sliced pitted black olives
- Canned or jarred artichoke hearts, sliced
- Sliced oil-packed sun-dried tomatoes

FEELING GREEN: Take this pesto from green to white: Omit the basil and reduce the olive oil to ¼ cup plus 1 tablespoon. Heat the 1 tablespoon of olive oil in a small pan over medium heat. Chop the garlic, add to the pan, and sauté until tender, about 3 minutes. Proceed with the recipe as directed.

FEELING FOOD: My mom, Tami, is a master entertainer, and this is one of her favorite shortcuts because it gets a "wow" reaction from guests every time.

Prepare the pesto sauce. Heat 1 tablespoon of oil in a skillet over medium heat. Add 2 crushed garlic cloves and 2 tablespoons of chopped basil, and sauté for 3 minutes. Add 1 cup of cream and heat until just before boiling. Drizzle the cream into the pesto sauce, stirring gently. Pour over a pound of your favorite pasta, cooked, and serve hot or at room temperature. Alternatively, try serving Sun-Dried Tomato Pesto (recipe follows) over pasta and top with fresh goat cheese.

FEELING FULL: Preparing a vinaigrette from the pesto will allow you to enjoy its aromatic flavors without using quite as much, and to serve it over greens instead of pasta. Prepare the pesto as directed. (You may want to make only half the recipe.) In a small bowl or cup, whisk together 3 tablespoons of the pesto with 2 teaspoons of balsamic vinaigrette and 1 teaspoon of water. Use as a vinaigrette over your favorite salad, and store in the refrigerator (will keep for 2 weeks).

Sun-Dried Tomato Pesto • MAKES 1 CUP

Try this variation of classic pesto when you want an earthier, more robust flavor that holds its own when served over pasta as a side to steak or any other red meat.

>   1 cup sun-dried tomatoes (dry-packed, not oil-packed)
>   1 small clove garlic, crushed
>   2 tablespoons freshly grated Parmesan cheese
>   ¼ cup extra-virgin olive oil
>   ¼ cup chopped fresh Italian parsley

Put the tomatoes in a bowl. Bring 1 cup of water to a boil and pour over the tomatoes. Let soak for 20 minutes. Drain the tomatoes and pat dry.

In the bowl of a food processor, blend the tomatoes, garlic, and cheese to a rough paste. Add olive oil, blend until smooth, add the parsley, and pulse to combine. The pesto can be kept in an airtight container, refrigerated, up to 2 weeks.

Fettuccine with Mushrooms and Slow-Roasted Tomatoes

• SERVES 4

With its earthy flavors, this dish speaks of fall, but it is so delicious, you may want to make it year-round. According to Chinese medicine, pregnancy and postpartum can cause "weak blood," a yin condition. Treatment requires yang foods that are high in blood-building properties. Mushrooms are one of these foods. The darker the mushroom, the more blood-building it is, so consider shiitakes or creminis for this sauce, rather than their lighter cousin, the button mushroom. Slow-roasted tomatoes add magic to any dish. Keep in mind that roasting them takes about 1½ hours.

8 ounces dried fettuccine, penne, or fusilli

2 tablespoons olive oil

2 medium shallots, sliced

8 ounces mixed mushrooms, trimmed and sliced

2 teaspoons chopped fresh thyme

½ cup dry white wine or chicken or vegetable stock,
     homemade (page 66 or 67) or store-bought

1 cup Slow-Roasted Tomatoes (recipe follows), chopped

2 tablespoons chopped fresh Italian parsley

Salt and freshly ground pepper

Extra-virgin olive oil, if needed

Freshly grated Parmesan cheese for garnish

Cook the pasta according to package directions. Drain and transfer to a large mixing bowl.

Meanwhile, heat the olive oil in a large skillet over medium-high heat. Add the shallots and sauté for 1 minute. Add the mushrooms and, stirring frequently, cook until all the liquid has evaporated and the mushrooms turn a beautiful golden brown, about 10 minutes.

Add the thyme, increase the heat to high, and add the wine. Cook until the liquid evaporates, about 2 minutes. Add the roasted tomatoes and heat through, 1 or 2 minutes.

Add the pasta to the sauce along with half the parsley, season with salt and pepper, and toss to coat. If it seems a little dry, add a drizzle of extra-virgin olive oil. Serve immediately, topped with the remaining parsley and the Parmesan cheese.

FEELING GREEN: Some claim that slow-cooking tomatoes breaks down the acidity (others claim it brings it out further because of the water that is lost). So this one depends on how you are feeling about tomatoes these days. If you do try out the dish, be generous with the Parmesan topping, to balance the acidity.

FEELING FOOD: When adding the roasted tomatoes, add ½ cup of heavy cream and bring to a boil. Cook for 1 minute and then toss with pasta for a beautiful, creamy mushroom and tomato sauce.

FEELING FULL: Skip the pasta and prepare a beautiful roasted tomato with goat cheese salad. While the roasted tomatoes are cooling, toss 1 cup mixed greens with 1 tablespoon Sherry Vinaigrette (page 73). Place on a plate and top with 3 roasted tomato quarters in the center. Lay a thinly sliced medallion of Boucheron or another fresh goat cheese on top—and enjoy!

Slow-Roasted Tomatoes • MAKES ABOUT 2 CUPS

Slow roasting concentrates the flavor of tomatoes while mellowing their acidity. Serve them as an unexpected (and oh, so easy) side to seared chicken, beef, and tofu. Double up on the recipe and store in the refrigerator for quick meals.

    ¼ cup olive oil
     4 cloves garlic, minced
     1 tablespoon dried herbes de Provence, or 1 tablespoon chopped fresh
            rosemary plus 2 tablespoons chopped fresh thyme, or ½ teaspoon dried
            rosemary plus 1 teaspoon dried thyme
    12 plum tomatoes (about 2 pounds), quartered
        Salt and freshly ground pepper

Preheat the oven to 300°F.

Combine oil, garlic, and herbs in a baking dish, add the tomatoes, and toss until evenly coated. Season lightly with salt and generously with pepper. Roast in the oven until the tomatoes are very soft and have begun to shrivel, about 1½ hours.

If not using immediately, cool completely before storing in an airtight container. The tomatoes will keep for 1 week in the refrigerator.

Vegetarian Three-Bean Chili • SERVES 6 TO 8

Married to a vegetarian for eight years now, my husband, Dori, has had to eat his share of meatless chilies and declared this one to be his hands-down favorite. "Something about the earthy mix of spices and flavors made me feel like this is an authentic chili, like what cowboys used to eat around the fire," he said.

Don't let the long list of ingredients fool you—preparing this dish is actually quick and easy. Just factor in the 1-hour simmering time. Chili also improves vastly when made in advance. Keep it in the fridge for up to 2 days or freeze it for up to 1 month.

3 tablespoons olive oil
1 medium sweet onion, chopped
1 medium carrot, chopped
2 jalapenos, seeded and minced
1 medium green, red, or yellow bell pepper, chopped, optional
4 cloves garlic, minced
2 tablespoons chile powder
1½ teaspoons ground cumin
1 teaspoon ground coriander
1 teaspoon paprika
1 (15-ounce) can black beans, rinsed and drained
1 (15-ounce) can red beans, rinsed and drained
1 (15-ounce) can white beans, rinsed and drained
2 (16-ounce) cans crushed tomatoes, with their juice
1 sprig fresh thyme
1 bay leaf
½ teaspoon dried oregano
1 (12-ounce) bottle dark beer, preferably Mexican, or 1½ cups water
Salt and freshly ground pepper

Heat the olive oil in a heavy-bottomed, large saucepan over medium heat. Add the onion, carrot, jalapeños, and bell pepper and cook until the onion is translucent, about 5 minutes. Add the garlic, chili powder, cumin, coriander, and paprika and cook for 1 minute to bring out their flavors. The spices may stick to the pan; this is fine, just keep stirring.

Add the beans, tomatoes and their juice, thyme, bay leaf, oregano, and beer, and bring to a boil. Cover, reduce the heat, and simmer for 1 hour.

Season with salt and pepper, and discard the thyme and bay leaf before serving.

FEELING GREEN: Don't do it. Chili is hard enough to digest under any circumstance, but when you are feeling green it can really send your delicate system into a tizzy! If you are in the mood for some beans, try the Feeling Green variation of Stewed Lentils and Rice (page 136) or Italian Lentil Soup (page 56) for a gentler version of a warm, vegetarian, protein-filled meal.

FEELING FOOD: Add some browned ground turkey for a heartier version of this nourishing dish. Top with some shredded cheddar. Yum!

FEELING FULL: This high-protein, fiber-rich dish ensures that very little will take you quite far. Enjoy with a large salad for a satiating meal.

ABOUT BEANS

Some people call beans the perfect food. Here is why: They are high in vitamins B, K, folate, calcium, iron, magnesium, and potassium. They contain loads of dietary fiber, are an excellent source of complex carbohydrates, and stabilize blood sugar levels. Beans are heart healthy and rich in antioxidants, they lower cholesterol, and they are economical and easy to make.

LEGEND HAS IT . . .

According to Cherokee Indian lore, mothers who wanted their brood to look happy would take beans that cracked open in cooking and rub them over their children's lips, hoping to impart the smile shape of the beans to the children's mouths.

Stewed Lentils and Rice • SERVES 2

Almost every culture has its own take on stewed beans and rice, featuring red beans in Haiti and Louisiana, black beans in Latin America, and chickpeas in Africa. Pick your favorite legume for this recipe to make your very own version of this flavorful dish, which has a little kick in each bite. Because they require no soaking, lentils are easy to cook, but if you want to skip that first cooking step, just rinse and drain one 15-ounce can of your favorite beans and add to the skillet when adding the tomato.

1 cup dried lentils
1 bay leaf, optional
1 tablespoon olive oil
1 small shallot, chopped
1 clove garlic, minced
½ jalapeño, seeded and minced
 Pinch of ground cumin
1 medium tomato, seeded and chopped
1 tablespoon chopped scallions, white and green parts
 Salt and freshly ground pepper
2 cups cooked rice (see page 173)
1 tablespoon chopped fresh cilantro

Combine the lentils with 2 cups of water and the bay leaf in a medium saucepan and bring to a boil over high heat. Reduce the heat and simmer, partially covered, until the lentils are soft, 25 to 30 minutes. Drain if necessary.

Heat the oil in a large skillet over medium-high heat. Add the shallot, garlic, and jalapeño, and sauté for 2 to 3 minutes. Add the cumin, stir once, and then add the tomato and lentils. Simmer for 5 minutes, adding a little water if the lentils seem dry.

Stir in the scallions, season with salt and pepper, and serve over the rice, garnished with cilantro.

FEELING GREEN: The rule of thumb is smaller is better for digestion, so go with lentils as your legume of choice. Omit the jalapeño but otherwise, prepare as directed and enjoy with plain, brown rice.

FEELING FOOD: Try this out with a red bean or kidney bean over basmati rice. Top with 1 table-spoon of sour cream for a hot-and-cold contrast.

FEELING FULL: Enjoy your choice of bean over steamed quinoa or millet (see page 173) instead of rice.

Stir-Fried Vegetables with Coconut Curry Sauce • SERVES 2

Beware: this stir-fry is downright addictive. With its smooth and flavorful sauce, crunchy vegetables, and indescribably fresh taste, it may discourage you from ever ordering a take-out stir-fry again. Serve this delicious dish over rice, noodles, or quinoa. You can find curry paste at Asian markets or in health food stores.

1½ teaspoons canola oil

2 teaspoons peeled and grated fresh ginger

1 clove garlic, minced

4 ounces green beans, trimmed and cut on the diagonal into 1½-inch pieces

2 cups broccoli florets

1 medium carrot, peeled and cut into matchsticks

½ cup vegetable stock, homemade (page 67) or store-bought

1 teaspoon sweet or hot curry paste

¾ cup canned coconut milk

Salt and freshly ground pepper

2 tablespoons chopped scallions, white and green parts

2 tablespoons chopped roasted peanuts, optional

½ cup fresh cilantro leaves

In a large skillet heat the oil over medium-high heat. Add ginger and garlic and cook for 1 minute. Add the green beans, broccoli, carrot, and stock, cover the pan, and cook until the beans and broccoli have turned bright green, 1 to 2 minutes.

Stir the curry into the coconut milk. Increase the heat under the skillet to high and add the curry mixture to the vegetables. Cook, stirring often, until the vegetables are crisp-tender, 3 to 4 minutes more. Add salt and pepper to taste and stir in the scallions.

Sprinkle with chopped nuts and cilantro leaves before serving.

FEELING GREEN: Replace the green beans with 1 cup of sliced mushrooms and the broccoli with 2 cups of sliced zucchini. Select a sweet curry paste and increase the cooking time to 5 minutes, until the vegetables are very tender. Enjoy over a bed of basmati rice.

FEELING FOOD: This fabulous stir-fry works well with shrimp, chicken, or seared tofu (see page 138). Add your favorite protein and serve over a bed of soba noodles.

FEELING FULL: Add some chopped kale for extra nutrients. Reduce the coconut milk to ½ cup and the curry to ½ teaspoon.

Seared Tofu and Vegetables with Soy, Ginger, and Red Chiles • SERVES 2

This feisty stir-fry gets a kick from the fresh ginger, garlic, and chile. It works just as well with a wide range of veggies as it does with a single head of broccoli. This method of searing the tofu has had some of our most adamant antitofu clients clamoring for more.

1 pound extra-firm tofu

Salt and freshly ground pepper

1 tablespoon canola oil

2 teaspoons toasted sesame oil

1 tablespoon peeled and grated fresh ginger

1 clove garlic, minced

3 cups mixed vegetables, such as broccoli florets, green beans, carrots, asparagus, or yellow squash, cut into 2-inch pieces

1 teaspoon sambal (see page 81) or another ground chile paste

½ cup vegetable stock, homemade (page 67) or store-bought

2 tablespoons reduced-sodium tamari or soy sauce, or to taste

1 cup steamed brown or basmati rice (see page 173) or cooked soba noodles

2 tablespoons chopped scallions, white and green parts

1 tablespoon sesame seeds, preferably a mix of black and white

Cut the tofu in half lengthwise and wrap each piece in paper towels. Place on a plate and put another plate on top. Weigh down with canned tomatoes or beans for 30 minutes to remove excess moisture.

Pat the tofu dry and season with salt and pepper. Heat 2 teaspoons of oil in a heavy-bottomed skillet over medium-high heat. Sear the tofu blocks until crisp and golden brown, 3 to 4 minutes per side. Remove to a cutting board and let cool slightly. Cut each block into 8 pieces: first cut into quarters, and then cut each quarter in half diagonally to form triangles. Set aside.

Add the remaining teaspoon of oil to the skillet along with the sesame oil and heat over medium-high heat. Add the ginger and garlic, sauté for 1 minute, and then add the vegetables. Mix together the sambal and stock and add to the pan. Increase the heat to high, cover the pan, and cook the vegetables until the broccoli is bright green, 1 to 2 minutes.

Add the tamari and tofu. Cook, stirring constantly, until the vegetables are crisp-tender and the tofu is coated with sauce and heated through, 1 to 2 minutes.

To serve, place a mound of rice on each plate or shallow bowl. Arrange the tofu triangles in a circle around the rice, top with vegetables, and sprinkle with scallions and sesame seeds. Serve immediately, passing extra tamari on the side if desired.

FEELING GREEN: Choose vegetables that work well for you, even if it means using 3 cups of the same kind. Skip the chile paste and increase the cooking time to 3 to 4 minutes, until the vegetables are very tender. Enjoy over a bed of basmati rice.

FEELING FOOD: Omit the chile paste and tamari and add ¾ cup of coconut milk mixed with 1 teaspoon of sweet curry paste along with the tofu. Enjoy over a bed of soba noodles.

FEELING FULL: This delicious, nutritious stir-fry works well on its own or over a bed of quinoa or millet (see page 173).

REAL WORLD

It was delicious! I really liked the mixture of spices and how they flavored the food. Frankly, when making vegetarian food, we often neglect to use much in the way of spice, and so sometimes our dishes, while tasting wholesome, do taste a bit bland. In this case, the ginger and soy really made for a nice combination. Our local supermarket didn't carry sambal or ground chile paste, so, my husband, Jonathon (who made the meal—I really can't take credit!), simply substituted red pepper flakes. We chose to use asparagus, carrots, and broccoli as our vegetable ingredients, and they worked really nicely together. Our four-year-old, Christian, was intrigued enough to ask to try the tofu! While he didn't care for it (he actually used typical four-year-old vernacular to convey those feelings), we did congratulate him on trying a new food. Christian did ask if the baby inside me liked the food, and I assured him that the baby did like the food very much!

Lynn Miller, Bethesda, MD

Marinated Tofu and Vegetable Kebabs • SERVES 4

Although you can make this under your broiler, these kebabs are great backyard grilling fare. A soak in the marinade gives the tofu a delicious tangy twist and depth of flavor, and its grilled taste rivals that of its meat counterparts. Serve the kebabs with the Brown Rice Pilaf with Citrus and Toasted Almonds (page 162) and a beautiful summer salad such as the Provençal Carrot Salad (page 88) to enhance the sweetness of the marinade.

When considering your prep time, take into account that draining the tofu takes 30 minutes and marinating it another 3 hours. If using wooden skewers, be sure to soak them in water for 15 to 30 minutes before threading the ingredients onto them to prevent the wood from burning.

1 pound extra-firm tofu
1/2 cup reduced-sodium tamari or soy sauce
2 tablespoons fresh orange juice
1 tablespoon peeled and grated fresh ginger
1 tablespoon toasted sesame oil
1 teaspoon sambal (see page 81) or other ground chile paste, optional
Pinch of freshly ground pepper
8 leaves collard greens, kale, or Swiss chard, stems and center veins removed
2 medium red onions, cut into 2-inch chunks
2 small yellow squash, cut into 1-inch chunks
1 pint cherry tomatoes

Cut the tofu in half lengthwise and wrap each piece in paper towels. Place on a plate and put another plate on top. Weigh down with canned tomatoes or beans for 30 minutes to remove excess moisture.

Cut the tofu into 1½-inch chunks. In a shallow baking dish, mix the tamari, orange juice, ginger, oil, sambal, if using, and pepper. Add the tofu and stir to coat well. Refrigerate for at least 3 hours or overnight.

Boil the collard leaves and onions in a pot full of boiling water for 2 minutes (if using Swiss chard, 1 minute will do). Drain in a colander and run cold water over them to stop the cooking; then pat dry. Fold the leaves to make 1½-inch-square packages.

Prepare a medium-hot fire in a charcoal grill, preheat a gas grill to medium-high, or preheat the broiler.

Remove the tofu from the marinade with a slotted spoon, and toss the onions and squash in the marinade. Thread the tofu and vegetables on skewers, alternating colors. Brush the kebabs with any remaining marinade, and grill until the vegetables are cooked and the tofu is a deep golden brown, 3 to 4 minutes on each side.

FEELING GREEN: If the thought of tofu makes you queasy, marinate a thin piece of chicken breast instead. Replace the greens and onion with 8 ounces each of mushrooms and asparagus.

FEELING FOOD: Turn this marinade into a delicious soy-ginger glaze: increase the tamari to ¾ cup, replace the orange juice with ¼ cup of honey, and increase the sesame oil to 1½ tablespoons. Prepare as directed.

FEELING FULL: Skip the grill and the tofu. Dip your favorite fish in the marinade and broil. Enjoy with Asian Cabbage Salad (page 80).

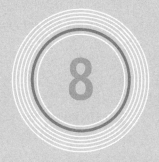

8

❈ Vegetables

We already know that what you feed your child as a toddler goes a long way in developing his future tastes. But recent research theorizes that this process begins even earlier—that a child's taste buds begin to develop in utero and while nursing. What better motivation to eat your vegetables now than knowing that you are creating a foundation for a healthy eater who has a taste for them later. Picture this: "Mommy, can I have some salad, please?" It happens!

The key to maximizing the benefits of eating your vegetables is color. Every vegetable color represents different vitamins, minerals, and other requirements for your body. If you can incorporate at least one serving of leafy greens (such as kale, spinach, bitter greens, and broccoli) along with two to three colorful vegetables in your daily routine, you will be building an excellent nutritional foundation for yourself and your children. Let me say here that when you are feeling green, the last thing you may want are your greens (see Lauren's story on page 17)! That is why many of the Feeling Green or Feeling Food variations that follow incorporate vegetables into other dishes, such as vegetable pancakes (see page 154). These are a great way to serve children their vegetables as well, in case the researchers are a little off base, and your baby isn't begging for broccoli.

Spinach, Pine Nuts, and Golden Raisins • SERVES 2

Eating your greens has never been more delicious than with this classic Italian recipe, which features wilted spinach, sweet raisins, and crunchy toasted pine nuts. But if you are not up for it, check out the Feeling Green and Feeling Food variations below for creamy spinach soup and creamed spinach.

> 1 tablespoon extra-virgin olive oil
> 1 small shallot, sliced very thin
> 1 (5-ounce) bag baby spinach
> 2 tablespoons golden raisins
> Salt and freshly ground pepper
> 2 tablespoons pine nuts, toasted (see page 70)

Heat the olive oil in a large skillet over medium heat. Add the shallot and cook until tender, about 2 minutes. Add the spinach and raisins, and stir constantly until the spinach is just wilted, about 2 minutes. Season with salt and pepper, sprinkle with pine nuts, and serve.

FEELING GREEN: Turn your spinach into a creamy soup. Omit the raisins and pine nuts. Use a medium pot and add ½ cup of chicken or vegetable stock, homemade (page 66 or 67) or store-bought, when you add the spinach. Simmer until the spinach is just wilted, 3 to 4 minutes. Puree the soup with an immersion blender. Add another ½ cup of stock along with 2 tablespoons of heavy cream and bring to a simmer. Add 1 tablespoon of lemon juice and salt and freshly ground pepper to taste. This recipe will yield 2 (1-cup) servings.

FEELING FOOD: Omit the raisins and pine nuts. Just as the spinach begins to wilt, stir in 2 tablespoons of cream cheese for a lighter take on popular creamed spinach.

FEELING FULL: Though pine nuts and raisins are pretty caloric, they give a high rate of return in nutrients and satisfaction levels. When you are in the mood for something sweet and crunchy, but don't want to give up on your intentions of lightening up, this is the perfect dish.

Sugar Snap Peas with Tomato and Mint • SERVES 4

The 1970s introduced us to a spectrum of creations ranging from bell-bottoms to the first test-tube baby. It is also the decade that brought sugar snap peas to the American dinner table. A cross between snow peas and garden peas, sugar snaps are sweet and should live up to their name: fresh sugar snaps should be crisp enough to snap when you bend them in half. Like all peas, they are filled with vitamin K, folic acid, and B6. Eaten raw, sugar snaps make a fabulous snack; simply remove the strings, wash, and dry well. Store in a bowl in the fridge for a quick snack, or chop them up and add to your salad. This 5-minute recipe takes them to the next level.

1 tablespoon olive oil

1 large shallot, minced

8 ounces sugar snap peas, stems and strings removed

2 large plum tomatoes, seeded and chopped into uniform small dice

2 tablespoons thinly sliced fresh mint

Salt and freshly ground pepper

Heat the olive oil in a large skillet over medium-high heat. Add the shallot and cook for 1 minute. Add the sugar snaps and sauté, stirring frequently, until the peas turn bright green, 2 to 3 minutes. Add the tomatoes, cook for 1 minute, and add the mint. Stir quickly to wilt the mint. Season with salt and pepper to taste and serve immediately.

In a pinch: Any sweet herb, such as tarragon, basil, or dill, can be substituted alone or in combination for the mint. And if sugar snaps are unavailable, substitute with their horticultural forbears, snow peas (the smaller, the sweeter).

FEELING GREEN: Although the mint in this recipe may be helpful, peas can cause bloating, which can increase nausea. Try out the Feeling Green variation of the Sautéed Zucchini and Yellow Squash with Baby Tomatoes and Dill (page 154) instead.

FEELING FOOD: Chop the sugar snaps before adding to the skillet, and then prepare the recipe as indicated. Stir the mixture into 2 cups of cooked basmati or brown rice.

FEELING FULL: Enjoy a bowl of this as a snack or as a side dish to your favorite entree, such as Grilled Chicken with Summer Salsa (page 118) or Broiled Halibut Provençal (page 110).

Balsamic-Glazed Beets • SERVES 2

Some women report cravings for beet juice during pregnancy; this may actually be the body's way of asking for more folate, which beets are full of, along with magnesium, potassium, and dietary fiber. Beets are also excellent for digestion and help to prevent anemia. Their sweet flavor is partly due to their high sugar content and is balanced by the vinegar in this delicious dish.

Note that beet juice can stain your hands. You can wear gloves when working with them or rub your hands with lemon juice to remove the red color. You can also replace fresh beets with canned.

4 medium beets, each about 2½ inches in diameter
1 tablespoon extra-virgin olive oil
1 medium shallot, thinly sliced
1 tablespoon balsamic vinegar
  Salt and freshly ground pepper

Bring 1 or 2 inches of water to a boil in the bottom of a steamer or a medium pot fitted with a steamer insert. Trim the stem and root ends of the beets and peel with a paring knife. Cut into ½-inch-thick wedges. Place the beets in the basket in an even layer. Cover and steam over medium heat until tender, about 10 minutes.

Heat the olive oil in a large skillet over medium-high heat. Add the shallot, and cook for 1 minute. Add the beets and vinegar, stir well, and cook until the vinegar has evaporated and the beets are glossy, about 2 minutes. Season with salt and pepper to taste and serve hot, at room temperature, or cold.

FEELING GREEN: The balance of sweet and sour of this recipe may make it your new favorite vegetable dish.

FEELING FOOD: My husband, who is of Russian heritage, finds great delight in this smooth borscht. Trim and peel the beets as directed, but do not slice; instead, grate them with a food processor or box grater. Chop 1 medium carrot, 1 celery stalk, and 1 medium shallot. Heat 1 tablespoon of olive oil in a large soup pot. Add the beets, carrot, celery, and shallot, and cook until softened, about 5 minutes. Add 4 cups of vegetable stock, homemade (page 67) or store-bought, and bring to a boil. Reduce the heat and simmer, covered, for 20 minutes. Add 1 tablespoon of lemon juice and season with salt and pepper to taste. Enjoy hot or chilled, topped with a dollop of sour cream, of course. This makes about 1½ quarts or 3 to 4 servings.

FEELING FULL: These delicious beets will enhance any salad. Simply layer over baby greens with a little goat cheese and a tablespoon of walnuts for a delicious, nutritious mini-meal.

Sautéed Kale • SERVES 4

If any single vegetable deserves the title of superfood, it would be kale. One serving of kale will supply you with more than the recommended intake of vitamin A, 88 percent of your daily requirement of vitamin C, and as much calcium as half a glass of milk. (In fact, some say that kale's calcium is better absorbed by the body.) This Mothers & Menus staple is a simple, tasty way to enjoy kale with minimal effort and maximum benefit. This method of cooking kale has you eating it at just the right level of doneness, but if you are new to the vegetable, you may want to leave it in the pot for another 2 minutes, to make it a little more tender.

1 pound kale (about 1 bunch), stems and center veins removed, leaves cut into 1-inch-wide strips
1½ tablespoons extra-virgin olive oil
1 large shallot, thinly sliced
¼ cup chicken or vegetable stock, homemade (page 66 or 67) or store-bought, or water
Salt and freshly ground pepper

Bring 1 or 2 inches of water to a boil in the bottom of a steamer or a medium pot fitted with a steamer insert. Add the kale, cover the steamer, and steam until the kale is tender, about 4 minutes.

In a large skillet, heat the olive oil over medium-high heat. Add the shallot and cook for 2 minutes, add the kale and stock and cook until the stock has evaporated and the kale is tender, about 2 minutes. Season with salt and pepper to taste and serve.

FEELING GREEN: Bring a large pot of water to a boil for some pasta, and prepare the kale as directed; the shallot is optional. Add 8 ounces of penne or fusilli to the boiling water and cook according to the package directions. While the pasta is cooking, add ½ cup of ricotta and ½ cup of grated Parmesan cheese to the kale and mix. When the pasta is ready, drain and add it to the kale mixture. Toss well and enjoy.

FEELING FOOD: Try the Feeling Green variation.

FEELING FULL: Have a serving of kale every day and you will not be feeling full for long. Its fiber and nutrients will help your digestive system process the other foods that you are eating, and it will also keep you feeling satiated and balance out your food cravings. Accompany with a piece of broiled fish (try Broiled Halibut Provençal, page 110) or seared tofu (see page 138) and a serving of your favorite whole grain for a perfectly balanced meal.

Broccoli with Garlic and Lemon • SERVES 4

Broccoli comes alive with a hint of garlic and a burst of lemon here. This dish is Italian all the way, and a prime example of how spectacular simple can be.

1 pound broccoli (about 1 medium head)
1 tablespoon olive oil
2 cloves garlic, minced
½ cup chicken or vegetable stock, homemade
    (page 66 or 67) or store-bought
½ teaspoon red chile flakes, optional
1 lemon, cut into wedges
    Salt and freshly ground pepper

Cut the broccoli into 3-inch florets. Peel the tough skin from the remaining stems and slice into ¼-inch-thick coins.

Heat the olive oil in a large heavy skillet over medium-high heat. Add the garlic and cook for 1 minute. Add the broccoli, stock, and chile flakes. Stir, cover the pan, and cook for 2 minutes. Increase the heat to high, squeeze in 2 tablespoons of lemon juice, and continue to cook, covered, until the broccoli is crisp-tender, about 2 minutes. Season to taste with salt and pepper and serve immediately, garnished with lemon wedges.

FEELING GREEN: This lemony dish may become your new way of preparing all your greens. Omit the chile flakes and leave the broccoli on the stove for 2 minutes more to soften further.

FEELING FOOD: Make with chicken stock and increase the amount to 1 cup. Cook the broccoli for an additional minute, and ladle the broccoli and broth over a bowl of cooked brown or basmati rice, sprinkled with toasted almonds.

FEELING FULL: Add this to Sesame Lotus Root Soba Noodles (page 167) with some diced tofu for a beautifully balanced meal.

REAL WORLD

This recipe was quick and easy to make, calling for ingredients that are usually lying in abundance around the house. My daughters, Amélie, four, and Chloé, two, love plain, steamed broccoli, but this was a welcome change for me and my husband, Jean-François. The only adaptation I made was to add another 3 minutes to the cooking time for the girls' portions, because it was too crunchy for their palates (I also eliminated the chile flakes). We have gotten so used to steaming broccoli for the kids that I forgot how good an adult version can be. This one is a keeper to try out with rapini (broccoli rabe) and broccolini as well.

Naomi Goldapple, Montreal, Canada

Green Beans with Carrots, Shallots, and Thyme • SERVES 4

Sweet shallots, crunchy carrots, and crisp green beans come together in a sophisticated twist on an old-fashioned favorite, giving a flavor boost to any entree.

1 pound green beans, stems removed

1 tablespoon extra-virgin olive oil

1 medium shallot, thinly sliced

1 medium carrot, peeled and cut into matchsticks

2 teaspoons minced fresh thyme

1/4 cup chicken or vegetable stock, homemade (page 66 or 67) or store-bought, or water

Salt and freshly ground pepper

Bring 1 or 2 inches of water to a boil in the bottom of a steamer or a medium pot fitted with a steamer insert. Add the green beans, cover the steamer, and steam until the beans are crisp-tender, about 3 minutes.

Heat the olive oil in a large skillet over medium heat. Add the shallot and cook for 2 minutes. Add the carrot and thyme, and sauté for 1 minute more. Add the green beans and stock, increase the heat, and cook, stirring constantly, until heated through, 1 to 2 minutes. Season with salt and pepper to taste and serve.

Express: No time to stem beans? Go for frozen green beans or French-cut beans, skip the steaming step, and go straight to sautéing the shallot.

FEELING GREEN: Try substituting haricots verts for the green beans. French green beans are thinner and smaller than their American counterparts and may be easier to digest. They can usually be found in farmers markets in summer. Omit the shallot and proceed as directed.

FEELING FOOD: For an updated green bean casserole, omit the carrots, thyme, and stock. Add 1 tablespoon of butter to the oil and sauté 2 shallots cut into rings. Increase the heat and cook, stirring frequently, until caramelized, 10 minutes. Add one 12-ounce package button mushrooms, wiped clean and thinly sliced. Cook over medium-high heat until the mushrooms are tender, about 5 minutes. Add the steamed beans, increase the heat, and cook, stirring, until heated through, 2 minutes. Serve with a generous sprinkling of grated Parmesan.

FEELING FULL: Enjoy this recipe as directed. Consider pairing with steamed millet (see page 173).

Roasted Winter Squash with Cinnamon and Nutmeg • SERVES 4

Honey, cinnamon, and nutmeg highlight squash's natural sweetness in this hearty, flavorful side, which welcomes fall with its warm, comforting spices. Any squash that appears at summer's end can be used for this: butternut, kabocha, acorn, buttercup, and pumpkin are all interchangeable here.

1 medium butternut squash, peeled, cut in half, seeded, and cut crosswise into ½-inch-thick slices

2 medium shallots, thinly sliced

1 tablespoon olive oil

2 tablespoons honey

1 teaspoon ground cinnamon

½ teaspoon ground ginger

Salt and freshly ground pepper

Preheat the oven to 400°F.

In a large bowl, toss the squash with the shallots, olive oil, honey, cinnamon, and ginger and season with salt and pepper. Spread out on a baking sheet in an even layer and roast until the squash is golden brown and tender, about 30 minutes. Serve hot or at room temperature.

FEELING GREEN: This recipe may prove too sweet. Tone it down by replacing the honey, cinnamon, and ginger with 1 tablespoon of chopped fresh thyme and 1 teaspoon of chopped fresh rosemary. Proceed as directed.

FEELING FOOD: After cooking as directed, transfer this squash to a blender or a large bowl. Using the blender, hand blender, or a masher, add 2 tablespoons of butter and blend into a distinctive, nutritious, flavorful mash.

FEELING FULL: Omit the honey and enjoy the squash's natural sweet flavors, or look to the Feeling Green variation for a savory take.

Sautéed Bitter Greens with Shallots • SERVES 2

Best prepared in the spring with young greens, this quick sauté is cleansing for the lymphatic system and liver, blood building, and a great overall tonic. A rich background of olive oil, garlic, and a hint of spice serve to enhance any green, including dandelion, collard, chard, and mustard.

1 tablespoon extra-virgin olive oil

1 large shallot, thinly sliced

2 cloves garlic, minced

½ teaspoon red chile flakes, optional

8 ounces young greens, such as mustard, dandelion, turnip, broccoli rabe, baby kale, or baby collards, stemmed and cut into ½-inch strips

½ cup chicken or vegetable stock, homemade (page 66 or 67) or store-bought

Salt and freshly ground pepper

Heat the olive oil in a skillet over medium-high heat. Add the shallot, garlic, and chile flakes, and cook, stirring constantly, for 2 minutes. Add the greens and stir for a minute to begin wilting them. Pour in the stock and cook until it has nearly evaporated and the greens are tender, about 4 minutes.

Season with salt and pepper to taste and serve with any remaining liquid from the pan, drizzled over the greens.

FEELING GREEN: Omit the shallot, garlic, and chile flakes. Arrange the warm greens on Bruschetta or Crostini (page 102) that has been drizzled with olive oil. Sprinkle with shredded Romano cheese and enjoy.

FEELING FOOD: Follow the Italian lead. Prepare as directed (remember, chiles are optional) and toss with 1 cup of pasta, such as penne or fusilli. Sprinkle with 2 tablespoons of grated Parmesan cheese.

FEELING FULL: Bitter greens are excellent for improved digestion and increased metabolism. Prepare as directed and consider Laurene's addition of tofu to the dish, or Richard's suggestion of using the pan juices to broil fish (see Real World, opposite).

REAL WORLD

I am always looking for something light but substantial and flavorful, but I hesitated to make this recipe because I thought it would take too much time. It literally took just minutes to prepare. I made it for my dad, Richard, and my husband, Will, alongside some whole wheat pasta. I used 4 medium shallots instead of the 1 called for. I love onions, scallions, and shallots—so for me, the more the better. I added tofu to my portion to make it a meal in itself.

Will and Dad both really enjoyed it, too. My dad suggested filling the bottom of a baking oven pan with the pan juices and broiling some fish in it, which sounded quite good. Will, of course, thought it would go best with a steak. As for William, age two, he ate the greens once I buried them in a bowl of mashed potatoes. I will definitely make this again as a quick and easy side dish for dinner.

Laurene Chavez, Long Island, NY

Sautéed Zucchini and Yellow Squash with Cherry Tomatoes and Dill • SERVES 4

Bright green zucchini, sunny yellow squash, and cherry red tomatoes are a joy to both the palate and the eye. Because zucchini have such a high water content, they produce a light dish that is great for the later days of pregnancy, when you just can't stomach heavy meals.

2 tablespoons olive oil

1 medium shallot, thinly sliced

2 small zucchini, cut into 1/2-inch rounds

2 small yellow squash, cut into 1/2-inch rounds

1 cup grape or cherry tomatoes, halved

2 teaspoons minced fresh dill

Salt and freshly ground pepper

2 teaspoons minced fresh chives

Heat the olive oil in a large skillet over medium-high heat. Add the shallot and cook for 1 minute. Add the zucchini and yellow squash and sauté, stirring frequently, until the squash is tender and beginning to turn golden, about 4 minutes. Add the tomatoes and dill and continue to cook, stirring constantly, for 1 minute. Season with salt and pepper to taste and serve immediately, garnished with chives.

FEELING GREEN: Roasting vegetables seems to make them more palatable. Preheat the oven to 425°F. Cut the zucchini and squash into 1-inch chunks. Omit the shallot, tomatoes, and chives. In a bowl, toss the zucchini and squash with the olive oil and dill and season with salt and pepper. Spread evenly on a baking sheet and roast for 15 minutes. Serve immediately.

FEELING FOOD: Turn these into vegetable pancakes. Using a food processor or box grater, grate the shallot, zucchini, and squash and place in a large bowl. Add 1 beaten egg and 5 tablespoons of whole wheat flour, along with the dill, chives, and some salt and pepper, and beat well. Omit the tomatoes. Heat the oil in a heavy skillet until very hot. Add tablespoonfuls of batter and cook until golden brown on both sides, about 6 minutes.

FEELING FULL: Go raw with this summer soup: Coarsely chop the zucchini, yellow squash, and shallot. In a blender, combine 1 clove of garlic, 3 cups of water, and 5 tablespoons of lemon juice, the zucchini, yellow squash, shallot, and dill and puree (you may have to do this in two batches). To serve, garnish the soup with tomatoes and chives. Enjoy immediately or chill for up to 1 day.

Roasted Asparagus with Lemon • SERVES 4

This simple recipe turns a healthy, nutrient-rich vegetable into an addictive, crunchy snack—so much so that when I first introduced them to Sophie, then three, she proclaimed them "asparagus chips" and now requests them often.

> 1 pound asparagus (1 bunch), tough stem ends removed
> 2 teaspoons extra-virgin olive oil
> Salt and freshly ground pepper
> Lemon wedges for serving

Preheat the oven to 450°F.

Scatter the asparagus on a baking sheet, drizzle with the olive oil, and season with salt and pepper. Toss gently to lightly coat the spears and spread out in a single layer. Roast until bright green and tender but al dente (firm to the bite), 10 minutes. Serve hot or at room temperature with lemon wedges.

FEELING GREEN: Use coarse salt on this dish and add a strong squeeze of lemon before enjoying this crunchy, salty, lemony preparation, which addresses most of your needs.

FEELING FOOD: Enhance this side dish with a creamy orange butter sauce: In a small saucepan, melt 2 tablespoons of butter over medium heat. Whisk in 2 teaspoons of fresh orange juice and 1 teaspoon of minced chives. Remove from the heat and drizzle over the asparagus.

FEELING FULL: Double up on this dish! Asparagus is a diuretic that will have you feeling less full in no time, and this method of preparation will surely satisfy.

Asian-Style Roasted Broccoli · SERVES 4 TO 6

Roasting broccoli with these Asian flavors adds a special something to this favorite green vegetable, so that you can enjoy it over and over again. Also, hold onto the Feeling Green version below as a simple yet tasty way to get your kids to eat their broccoli when they have outgrown the basic steamed variety.

1½ pounds broccoli (1 medium head), cut into 4-inch florets
2 cloves garlic, minced
1 medium shallot, minced
1 tablespoon peeled and chopped fresh ginger
1 tablespoon toasted sesame oil
1 tablespoon tamari or reduced-sodium soy sauce
Freshly ground pepper

Preheat the oven to 400°F.

In a bowl, mix the broccoli with the garlic, shallot, ginger, oil, and tamari and season with pepper to taste. Spread out in a single layer on a baking sheet and roast until the florets are tender but still bright green, about 20 minutes. Serve hot or at room temperature.

FEELING GREEN: Keep it simple for a milder version: omit the ginger and tamari, and replace the sesame oil with 2 tablespoons of olive oil. Proceed as directed, adding salt if needed.

FEELING FOOD: Turn this into a hearty meal by cooking one 8-ounce package of soba noodles according to the directions. Drain and transfer to a large bowl. Toss with 1 tablespoon of sesame oil, and then add 4 cups of diced cooked chicken and the Asian-Style Roasted Broccoli. Mix well and garnish with sesame seeds.

FEELING FULL: Up the nutrients on this by combining 1 tablespoon of tamari, 1 teaspoon of sesame oil, and 1 pound of extra-firm tofu, cubed, in a small bowl, and tossing everything together gently. Add to the broccoli mixture in the pan. Proceed with recipe as directed, and serve with 2 cups of cooked brown rice (see page 173).

Roasted Cauliflower with Curry • SERVES 4 TO 6

High in fiber, folate, water, and vitamin C, cauliflower is an excellent, nutrient-dense food, but it is often overlooked. Elevate the humble cauliflower to new heights with this Indian-inspired recipe, which combines sweet raisins, fragrant curry, and crunchy walnuts with a kick of ginger in every bite. You will never look down on cauliflower again.

½ cup dark raisins

¼ cup orange juice

1 pound cauliflower (about 1 head), cut into 2-inch florets

1 medium shallot, thinly sliced

1 tablespoon peeled and minced fresh ginger

1 cup walnut halves and pieces

1 tablespoon curry powder

1 teaspoon chopped fresh thyme

2 tablespoons olive oil

Salt and freshly ground pepper

Preheat the oven to 400°F.

In a large bowl, soak the raisins in the orange juice for 15 minutes. Add the cauliflower, shallot, ginger, walnuts, curry, thyme, and olive oil, season with salt and pepper, and mix well.

Spread out in a single layer on a baking sheet and roast until the florets are tender, about 20 minutes. Serve hot.

FEELING GREEN: Too many flavors may activate your nausea. Omit the orange juice, raisins, walnuts, and curry, and proceed with recipe as directed.

FEELING FOOD: Omit the walnuts, and bring this to the stovetop for a full-fledged Indian-style coconut curry. Soak the raisins. In a large saucepan, heat the olive oil over medium-high and add 1 medium peeled and diced Yukon Gold potato, along with the shallot and ginger. Cook, stirring constantly, for 5 minutes. Add the curry, thyme, and cauliflower along with ½ cup of cold water and 1 cup of coconut milk. Stir well. Bring to a boil, reduce the heat and simmer, covered, until the cauliflower and potato are tender, about 10 minutes. Stir in the soaked raisins, discarding the orange juice in which they soaked, and season with salt and pepper to taste. Serve immediately.

FEELING FULL: For a delicious entree salad, allow the cauliflower curry to cool and scoop 2 tablespoons onto 1 cup of loosely packed mixed greens, drizzled with Orange Vinaigrette (page 71).

Roasted Cremini Mushrooms with Herbs and Balsamic • SERVES 4

Mushrooms often evoke a love-it-or-leave-it reaction. Being a lover myself, I was thrilled to find out that mushrooms are very nutritious. Mushrooms provide a lot of iron, copper, and B2. Even better, none of this is lost in cooking. With a tangy taste of balsamic, these roasted mushrooms are meaty, juicy, and savory.

> 8 ounces cremini mushrooms
> 2 cloves garlic, minced
> 2 teaspoons chopped fresh thyme
> ½ teaspoon chopped fresh rosemary
> 1 tablespoon balsamic vinegar
> 1 tablespoon extra-virgin olive oil
> Salt and freshly ground pepper

Preheat the oven to 425°F.

In a medium bowl, toss together the mushrooms, garlic, thyme, rosemary, vinegar, and olive oil and season to taste with salt and pepper. Spread out on a baking sheet in a single layer and roast, shaking the pan midway through the cooking time to rotate the mushrooms, until they are tender, about 20 minutes. Serve hot or at room temperature.

FEELING GREEN: Chop the roasted mushrooms and add to a bowl of hot chicken or vegetable broth, homemade (page 66 or 67) or store-bought, along with some basmati rice for a soothing, nutrient-rich soup.

FEELING FOOD: Add the roasted mushrooms to cooked pasta, and add a drizzle of extra-virgin olive oil, some chopped parsley, and a generous sprinkling of Parmesan cheese.

FEELING FULL: While mushrooms are still hot, add them to baby spinach to gently wilt for a delicious warm salad. Top with Balsamic Vinaigrette (page 73) or Sherry Vinaigrette (page 73).

ABOUT CREMINIS

Cremini mushrooms are sometimes called "baby bellas" because when they are allowed to grow really wide, they become portobellos. In fact, portobellos were created in the 1980s, when farmers found a way to market overgrown, and at the time, unsalable, creminis.

Mediterranean Roasted Carrots and Parsnips • SERVES 4

With its combination of sweet orange juice and spicy mustard, this dish has a decidedly North African feel. Serve over a bed of whole wheat couscous, along with pan-seared chicken or fish. Pour the pan juices on top, sprinkle with some toasted slivered almonds (see page 70), and rent Casablanca *for the full effect.*

 5 medium parsnips, peeled and cut on the diagonal into 1-inch chunks
 5 medium carrots, cut on the diagonal into 1-inch chunks
 1 medium shallot, finely chopped
 1 teaspoon chopped fresh rosemary, or ½ teaspoon dried
 1 teaspoon mustard seeds
 ½ cup orange juice
 2 tablespoons extra-virgin olive oil
   Salt and freshly ground pepper

Preheat the oven to 400°F.

Toss the parsnips and carrots in a large bowl with the shallot, rosemary, mustard seeds, orange juice, and oil and season with salt and pepper. Spread out in a baking pan in an even layer and roast, stirring occasionally to coat the vegetables in the orange juice, until the vegetables are tender and golden brown, about 40 minutes. Serve hot or at room temperature.

FEELING GREEN: While the juice enhances the root vegetables' natural sweetness, it might be too acidic and sweet for you right now. So omit the orange juice and mustard seeds and add 1 tablespoon of chopped fresh thyme, or ½ teaspoon dried. Proceed with the recipe as directed.

FEELING FOOD: Go for a sweet, shiny glaze: Omit the mustard seeds, rosemary, and olive oil. Add 4 tablespoons of melted butter, ½ cup of pure maple syrup, and ½ teaspoon of ground cardamom, and proceed with recipe as directed. Serve with a simple roasted or broiled chicken.

FEELING FULL: With the natural sweetness of root vegetables, you can skip the sugar in the orange juice and follow the Feeling Green version. Serve with Broiled Salmon with Caramelized Fennel and Sweet Onion (page 108).

9

❖ Whole Grains, Potatoes & Other Starches

Ah, the poor, misunderstood carbohydrate—either overly indulged in or completely shunned. This chapter tries to find a happy medium by presenting you with choices: complex carbohydrates for most of the time, simple carbohydrates for some of the time, and some that fall in between for when you can't make up your mind (which might feel like all of the time).

Whole grains and refined starches all emanate from the same source. The difference is that while the whole grain remains intact, refined carbohydrates, such as white pasta and bread, are processed, which takes away their protein and fiber. The effect on your body is different, too. A refined or processed carbohydrate gives you an immediate blood sugar high, followed by a low, often accompanied with fatigue. A whole grain, on the other hand, enters your system slowly because it is accompanied by vitamins, minerals, fiber, and protein, leaving you feeling balanced. Of course, the processed carbohydrates have their job as well. The speed with which their sugar gets into the body provides a quick fix, and sometimes that is really what you need! If possible, it's best to try to balance those fixes with some vegetables and proteins to mitigate the sugar high. Or just have your pasta and enjoy it fully, switching over to a whole grain, such as quinoa or brown rice, for your next meal.

When it comes to potatoes, think of sweet potatoes as a whole grain and regular potatoes as a refined grain. Although regular potatoes come complete with their own vitamins and minerals, sweet potatoes bring a lot more to the table; they contain powerful antioxidants, are an excellent anti-inflammatory, and are helpful in stabilizing blood sugar. They also taste pretty amazing, proving that you can have your sweet and eat it too.

Brown Rice Pilaf with Citrus and Toasted Almonds • SERVES 2 TO 4

Light and brightly flavored, this pilaf works particularly well with fish and chicken entrees and grilled food such as Marinated Tofu and Vegetable Kebabs (page 140). The recipe can easily be multiplied for a crowd. Pumpkin seeds, pistachios, walnuts, pine nuts, cashews, or pecans can all be substituted for the almonds.

3 cups cooked long-grain brown basmati rice
(see page 173)
1 tablespoon olive oil
1 medium shallot, minced
¼ cup finely chopped carrot
1 tablespoon fresh lemon juice
2 tablespoons fresh orange juice
2 tablespoons chopped fresh Italian parsley
Salt and freshly ground pepper
¼ cup sliced almonds, toasted (see page 70)

Put the rice in a large serving bowl.

Heat the olive oil in a small skillet over medium heat. Add the shallot and carrot and sauté, stirring frequently, until softened, about 3 minutes. Add the lemon and orange juices and simmer to reduce slightly, about 1 minute.

Add the carrot mixture and the parsley to the rice and season with salt and pepper. Stir well and sprinkle with toasted almonds. Serve hot or at room temperature.

FEELING GREEN: This balanced dish may bring relief as well as much-needed protein and vegetables. Skip the shallot and add more parsley and lemon juice to taste. If you enjoy this mix, consider adding some lentils or garbanzo beans for an all-in-one dish.

FEELING FOOD: Replace the oil with 1 tablespoon of butter for a richer pilaf. Finish the rice with a sprinkling of dried cranberries or raisins for an extra sweet bite and uplifting color.

FEELING FULL: Reduce the oil to 1 teaspoon and omit the orange juice. Prepare as directed, but add 1 cup of chopped spinach in the last minute of sautéing the vegetables. Add ½ cup of cooked lentils to the rice. Sprinkle the dish with sliced raw almonds for a balanced bowl full of vegetables, protein, and complex carbohydrates.

The best thing about this rice pilaf recipe is its versatility: you can throw virtually *anything* into the mix! Because it's summer and we live near a farmers market, I decided to use only fresh ingredients that I could buy in season. I ended up with fresh onions, asparagus, and zucchini. Then I stopped at the supermarket and bought a precooked rotisserie chicken on the way home.

Instead of a saucepan, I used a rice cooker (same cooking time, but easier than a saucepan because you don't have to stir and it shuts off automatically when it's done). For some extra protein and flavor, I substituted organic, low-sodium chicken stock for the water. Once the rice was done, I threw it into a bowl, and then added the veggie-juice mixture, parsley, and shredded pieces of the rotisserie chicken. My baby can't eat nuts yet, but boy am I glad my husband insisted on toasting some almonds. We had them on our portions, and they were absolutely delicious—crunchy and fragrant.

This is a very easy recipe—the only real time-consuming thing is the chopping. But once it's done, you have enough for several days, and if you add chicken as we did, it really feels like a complete meal. If you're going for leftovers, I would use a different grain, like quinoa or whole wheat couscous—something that holds up better overnight.

This was a yummy recipe (amazing how much zip just a little bit of citrus juice adds), and I would definitely make it again.

Juliet Eastland, New York, NY

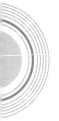

Quinoa with Mushrooms, Caramelized Squash, and Toasted Pecans • SERVES 4 TO 6

This recipe tastes and looks as delicious as it sounds. The sweet squash, earthy mushrooms, and crunchy pecans team together to enhance the protein-rich quinoa base, which is also an excellent source of magnesium, fiber, iron, and copper. This dish is a great way to introduce the grain to a newcomer.

3 cups cooked quinoa (see page 173)

2 tablespoons olive oil

6 ounces cremini mushrooms, stemmed and sliced

Salt and freshly ground pepper

1 small sweet onion, finely chopped

½ medium butternut squash, peeled, seeded, and cut into small dice

1 teaspoon chopped fresh thyme

½ cup pecans, toasted (see page 70) and chopped

Put the quinoa in a large serving bowl.

Heat 1 tablespoon of the oil in a large skillet over medium-high heat and sauté the mushrooms until brown, about 10 minutes. Season with salt and pepper and add to the quinoa.

Heat the remaining 1 tablespoon of oil in the skillet over medium-high heat. Add the onion and squash and cook, stirring frequently, until caramelized and golden brown, and the squash is cooked through, 10 to 12 minutes.

Add the thyme to the onions and squash and mix well. Stir the squash mixture into the quinoa and mushrooms. Mix well, taste, and adjust the seasonings with salt and pepper. Sprinkle with the pecans and serve hot.

FEELING GREEN: This balanced dish in a small dose may keep nausea at bay, while providing you with real nutrients.

FEELING FOOD: Add ½ cup of dried cranberries, currants, or raisins to elevate this sweet treat.

FEELING FULL: Once the squash is browned, add 1 cup of chopped spinach, stir briefly until the spinach is just wilted, and proceed with the recipe as indicated for a bowlful of basics: greens, grains, and proteins.

Basmati and Wild Rice Pilaf • SERVES 4 TO 6

Plain basmati goes wild with flavors and nutrition with the simple addition of wild rice, a grass seed that grows on tall reeds in shallow waters and small lakes. Wild rice is richer in protein and fiber than white or brown rice, and adds a depth of flavor that plays off the basmati for a splendid side to chicken or fish, such as Broiled Halibut Provençal (page 110), along with some greens, such as Asian-Style Roasted Broccoli (page 156).

3 cups cooked basmati rice (see page 173)
1 cups cooked wild rice (see page 173)
1 tablespoon butter
1 tablespoon olive oil
1 small sweet onion, finely chopped
1 medium carrot, peeled and finely chopped
1 medium leek, white part only, finely chopped
2 tablespoons chopped fresh Italian parsley
Salt and freshly ground pepper

Put the basmati rice and wild rice in a large serving bowl.

Melt the butter with the olive oil in a large skillet over medium heat. Add the onion, carrot, and leek and sauté until the vegetables are tender, about 8 minutes. Add the vegetables and parsley to the rice and season with salt and pepper to taste. Mix well and serve hot or at room temperature.

FEELING GREEN: Enjoy as is for a healthy take on rice and an opportunity to get in some vegetables.

FEELING FOOD: Sprinkle some toasted almonds over the rice for extra crunch.

FEELING FULL: Replace the basmati rice with brown rice to take this pilaf up one nutritional notch.

Orzo with Spinach, Lemon, Olive Oil, and Herbs • SERVES 4

This brightly flavored, satisfying side dish offers up a taste of summer, though it can easily be prepared all year long. Try it with Balsamic and Herb–Roasted Chicken (page 120) or any grilled chicken, fish, or tofu dish.

8 ounces orzo

2 tablespoons extra-virgin olive oil

1 medium shallot, minced

2 cloves garlic, minced

½ teaspoon grated lemon zest

1 tablespoon fresh lemon juice

1 (5-ounce) package baby spinach

Salt and freshly ground pepper

1 tablespoon chopped fresh Italian parsley

¼ cup freshly grated Parmesan cheese, optional

Cook the orzo according to the package directions and drain thoroughly. Transfer to a medium bowl.

Heat the oil in a large skillet over medium heat. Add the shallot, garlic, and zest and sauté for 2 minutes. Add the lemon juice, simmer for 1 minute, and then mix in the spinach. Cook just to wilt the greens, 1 minute.

Add the spinach mixture to the orzo and toss thoroughly. Season with salt and pepper to taste and sprinkle with parsley and Parmesan cheese, if desired, before serving—hot or at room temperature.

FEELING GREEN: The fresh lemon juice in this recipe may help you out, but the shallot and garlic may not, so please omit them. Add an additional tablespoon of parsley, to leverage its nausea-combating properties.

FEELING FOOD: Do not let the healthy ingredients fool you: this pasta dish is a great balance of comfort and healthy food. Prepare as directed, but add an extra tablespoon of Parmesan and toss while still hot for a warm and gooey dish.

FEELING FULL: Replace the orzo with 2 cups of cooked millet or quinoa (see page 173) and follow the recipe as directed for a side dish that allows you to pass on the refined carbs while keeping the protein, iron, and taste. Alternatively, add leftovers to chicken or vegetable stock to make a lovely, nourishing soup.

Sesame Lotus Root Soba Noodles • SERVES 4 TO 6

Lotus is rich in iron and vitamin B and C. Lotus root soba noodles are delicious, with a unique, earthy flavor. If you cannot find them (they are available in health food stores or Asian markets), use your favorite soba noodles in this simple, satisfying side dish.

1 (8-ounce) package lotus root soba noodles

4 ounces snow peas, trimmed and thinly sliced

1 medium carrot, peeled and cut into matchsticks

½ cup frozen shelled edamame, defrosted

1½ tablespoons toasted sesame oil

2 tablespoons low-sodium tamari or soy sauce

1 teaspoon sambal (see page 81) or another ground chile paste, optional

1 tablespoon black sesame seeds

1 scallion, green part only, thinly sliced

Cook the soba noodles according to the package directions, with one exception: during the last minute of cooking, add the snow peas, carrots, and edamame. Cook until the snow peas turn bright green, about 1 minute. Drain well, transfer to a large bowl, and toss with the oil, tamari, and sambal, if desired. Top with the sesame seeds and scallion before serving.

FEELING GREEN: Skip the sambal, but otherwise enjoy this noodle dish, and see if you can sneak in some small cubes of tofu for extra protein.

FEELING FOOD: Take this up a notch by preparing a creamy peanut butter sauce. Omit the sesame oil. In a small bowl, combine ½ cup of natural peanut butter, the 2 tablespoons of tamari or soy sauce, 1 tablespoon of raw sugar, the juice of ½ lime, and 1 minced garlic clove. Add ¼ cup of hot water and whisk well, adding more water as needed to make a creamy sauce. Taste and adjust the flavors, adding sambal for a spicier sauce. Toss with the soba and vegetables.

FEELING FULL: Unlike their white counterparts, soba noodles are a complex carbohydrate and can provide you with a lot of fuel, without the fatigue.

Herb-Roasted Potatoes • SERVES 2

Yukon Gold potatoes have a deep golden flesh and a rich, buttery flavor; Red Bliss potatoes are small and sweet. Either one will give exceptional results for this classic side dish.

12 ounces Yukon Gold potatoes or Red Bliss potatoes
1 teaspoon chopped fresh thyme
1/2 teaspoon chopped fresh rosemary
1 clove garlic, minced
1 1/2 tablespoons extra-virgin olive oil
Coarse salt and freshly ground pepper

Preheat the oven to 425°F.

Cut the Yukon Golds into 8 wedges each or Red Bliss into 4. In a bowl, toss the potatoes with the thyme, rosemary, garlic, and oil and season with salt and pepper.

Spread out in a single layer on a baking sheet, and roast, turning once or twice, until the potatoes are a deep golden brown and crispy, and tender when pierced with a fork, about 40 minutes. Serve hot.

FEELING GREEN: Salty foods help to keep nausea at bay, so enjoy this crispy side dish.

FEELING FOOD: Cut the potatoes into rectangular pieces about 1/2 inch thick for a french fry feel without the fried side effects.

FEELING FULL: Replace the Yukon Gold potatoes with sweet potatoes or try Crisp Roasted Sweet Potatoes (opposite).

Crisp Roasted Sweet Potatoes • SERVES 4

Sweet potatoes are extremely high in vitamin A and C, as well as vitamin B6. They are rich in antioxidants, are anti-inflammatory, and help stabilize blood sugar. The skins are very rich in nutrients, so try leaving them on. These potatoes are both incredibly easy to make and delicious beyond expectation. Crispy and sweet, they make a great side dish for highly seasoned dishes, whether meat, fish, or vegetarian.

4 medium sweet potatoes, with or without skins, cut into 2-inch wedges
2 medium shallots, thinly sliced
2 tablespoons olive oil
Coarse salt and freshly ground pepper

Preheat the oven to 400°F.

Toss the potato wedges with the shallots, olive oil, salt, and pepper. Spread out in a single layer on a baking sheet and roast for 35 to 40 minutes, until deep golden brown and crisp on the underside. Adjust the seasonings and serve.

FEELING GREEN: Prepare these without the shallots, but salt as much as you dare for a salty treat that will also get you thirsty for water.

FEELING FOOD: Prepare the recipe as directed and add a zingy dip: in a small bowl, mix ½ cup of sour cream, 1 tablespoon of chopped fresh chives or scallions (green parts), and 1 tablespoon of chopped mild green chiles (fresh or canned that have been drained and rinsed). Serve alongside the potatoes.

FEELING FULL: Sweet potatoes are low glycemic, an excellent complex carbohydrate, and a terrific, tasty treat that you can readily enjoy.

Miami-Style Ripe Plantains • SERVES 4

Plantains are rich in potassium and vitamin A, C, and B6; contain plenty of fiber; and are excellent for the digestive system. Their subtle sweetness and great meaty texture are delicious with everything from rice and beans to beef tenderloin. And they can, happily, be made without the excess oil sometimes seen in Latin restaurants. Here they are thinly sliced and sautéed in oil—not deep-fried.

For this recipe, look for ripe plantains, which have dark yellow skins streaked with black. Plantains have very thick skins, so cut off the tips, slice through the skin lengthwise with a small, very sharp knife, and gently peel back until the whole skin can be lifted off.

2 very ripe plantains, peeled
Coarse salt and freshly ground pepper
Canola oil for coating pan

Cut the plantains on the diagonal into ¼-inch slices. Season with salt and pepper.

Put enough oil in a large skillet just to coat the bottom and heat over medium-high heat. Add enough plantains to cover the bottom of the pan and cook until deep brown at the edges, about 1½ minutes per side.

Transfer to a plate lined with paper towels and season again with salt, if needed. Repeat with the remaining plantain slices. Serve hot, topped with Grilled Tomato Salsa (page 97).

FEELING GREEN: While these plantains contain less oil than their counterparts, they are still lightly fried and might not sit well with your stomach. Stick to grains for better results.

FEELING FOOD: Turn this into a spectacular dessert. Lightly salt the plantains before cooking (omit the pepper) and prepare as indicated. Serve with any of the following, or a combination: vanilla yogurt or ice cream, Dark Chocolate Glaze (page 185), chopped nuts, or shredded coconut.

FEELING FULL: Although rich in potassium and other nutrients, plantains are also high in sugar, so enjoy a small serving with your favorite Latin-style dish.

Potato and Celery Root Puree • SERVES 4

Rich in phosphorous and potassium, celery root (celeriac) adds a wonderful, subtle, earthy flavor to mashed potatoes and helps mitigate their simple-carb effect. Use Yukon Gold potatoes for a naturally buttery, golden finish.

2 medium Yukon Gold potatoes (about 12 ounces),
    peeled and cut into 2-inch chunks
1 medium celery root (about ³/₄ pound),
    peeled and cut into 1-inch chunks
½ cup milk
1 tablespoon butter
1 tablespoon chopped fresh chives
    Salt and freshly ground pepper, preferably white pepper

Put the potatoes and celery root in a large saucepan. Add enough salted cold water to cover by at least 1 inch and bring to a boil over high heat. Lower the heat and simmer until the potatoes and celery root are very tender when pierced with a knife, about 25 minutes.

Drain and return the vegetables to the saucepan. Keeping the pan over very low heat, mash the vegetables with a potato masher or hand-held mixer until smooth. Add the milk, butter, chives, and salt and pepper to taste. Serve hot.

FEELING GREEN: This creamy mix should work well for you. Start with ¼ cup of milk and 1 teaspoon of butter and then work your way up, so that the puree does not become too rich for your system.

FEELING FOOD: This dish is a classic comfort food, replenished with nutrients. Add soft roasted garlic (page 97) to enhance the flavors and kick it up a notch.

FEELING FULL: Prepare this puree using sweet potatoes in place of the Yukon Golds.

Creamless Potato Gratin • SERVES 4 TO 6

Think of this dish as gratin dauphinois (a rich French classic) goes to the spa and gets a makeover—one that leaves it shedding several pounds, and looking and feeling much better! This gratin has all of the "yum" factor minus the milk and cream of the original. It makes a hearty fall or winter dish and goes well with the Seared Beef Tenderloin with Port and Mushrooms (page 122) and a side of Sautéed Bitter Greens with Shallots (page 152).

1½ cups chicken or vegetable stock, homemade (page 66 or 67)
       or store-bought
1 clove garlic, peeled
4 teaspoons butter, melted, or olive oil
1 pound Yukon Gold potatoes (about 4 medium), peeled and thinly sliced
   Salt and freshly ground pepper
2 teaspoons chopped fresh thyme
¼ cup freshly grated Parmesan cheese

Preheat the oven to 350°F.

Bring the stock to a simmer and keep warm. Smash the garlic and rub it over the bottom and sides of an 8 × 8-inch baking dish. Brush the dish with 2 teaspoons of the butter. Layer the potatoes in the dish, seasoning each layer with salt, pepper, and a sprinkling of thyme. Pour the stock over the potatoes, pressing them down with a wooden spoon to submerge them in the stock.

Drizzle the potatoes with the remaining 2 teaspoons of butter and sprinkle with the Parmesan. Cover (aluminum foil is fine) and bake for 20 minutes. Uncover and bake until the potatoes feel tender when pierced with a knife and the top is golden brown, about 25 minutes. Serve hot.

FEELING GREEN: This lighter version of the rich original may work quite well for you.

FEELING FOOD: *Vive la France* for providing us with so many of our favorite comfort foods. Pay homage to the original: Preheat the oven to 425°F. Layer the potatoes with the following: 5 cloves of garlic, minced; salt and freshly ground pepper; and 1 cup of grated Emmenthal, Gruyère, or a similar cheese. Pour in 1½ cups of scalded milk (2 percent is okay, but skim milk will not work). Partially cover with foil, exposing some of the dish (so that the milk can evaporate). Bake for 30 minutes. Uncover and bake until the potatoes feel tender when pierced with a knife and the top is golden brown, 25 minutes.

FEELING FULL: Try the ultraspa version, replacing regular potatoes with sweet potatoes so that you are eating a complex carbohydrate that will keep you satiated longer.

Steamed Grains

Follow these simple instructions for basic grains to accompany any entree or vegetable. Most of the recipes call for 1 cup of the grain and will yield about 3 cups cooked. I've included wild rice here, too, because even though it isn't technically a grain—it's actually a grass—it is usually served like a grain. You'll notice that the recipe for wild rice calls for just ½ cup and makes 1½ cups: that's because it is best mixed with other grains before serving to balance its assertive flavor. Cooked grains keep well in the refrigerator for a few days or in the freezer for even longer. When reheating grains on a stovetop or in a microwave, add 1 to 2 tablespoons of water to allow them to steam.

Basmati Rice
In a medium saucepan, bring 2 cups of water or stock to a boil with a large pinch of salt. Add 1 cup of the rice. Stir, cover, and cook over very low heat for 20 minutes, until fluffy. Let stand, covered, for 10 minutes.

Long-Grain Brown Basmati Rice
In a medium saucepan, bring 2½ cups of water or stock to a boil with ¼ teaspoon of salt. Add 1 cup of the rice. Stir once, cover, and cook over very low heat for 40 minutes. Let stand, covered, for 5 to 10 minutes.

Wild Rice
In a small saucepan, bring 2 cups of water to a boil. Add ½ cup of wild rice, cover, and cook for 45 minutes, until the rice is fluffy and the kernels are cracked. Drain well. This yields 1½ cups.

Brown Rice
In a medium saucepan, bring 2½ to 3 cups of water or stock (the quantity depends on how moist you like your rice; adjust for preference) to a boil with a large pinch of salt. Add 1 cup of the rice. Stir, cover, and cook over very low heat for 45 minutes, until fluffy. Let stand, covered, for 10 minutes.

Millet
Bring 2 cups of water or stock to a boil (you can boil the water in your kettle). In a medium saucepan, heat 1 tablespoon of olive oil over medium-high heat. Add 1 cup of millet and toast for 1 minute. Add the water to the millet along with a large pinch of salt. Stir, cover, and cook over very low heat for 25 to 30 minutes, until fluffy. Let stand, covered, for 10 minutes.

Quinoa
In a medium saucepan, bring 2 cups of water or stock to a boil with a large pinch of salt; as an option, for a richer taste, add 1 tablespoon of olive oil. Add 1 cup of quinoa. Stir, cover, and cook over very low heat for 15 minutes, until fluffy. Let stand, covered, for 10 minutes.

Barley
In a medium saucepan, bring 2½ cups of water or stock to a boil with a large pinch of salt. If you like your barley super-soft, add just ½ cup of barley. If you prefer the chewier texture, add ¾ cup. Stir, cover, and cook over very low heat for 45 minutes. Let stand, covered, for 10 minutes.

10

Desserts

Oatmeal Raisin Cookies

Jam Dot Cookies

Two Lemon Cookies

Ultra-Energy Bar

Ricotta Cheesecake

Rich Chocolate Brownies

Devilicious Cupcakes

Fruit Crisp

Balsamic-Macerated Strawberries

Baked Apples with Nuts, Raisins, and Spices

Poached Peaches with Raspberries and Whipped Cream

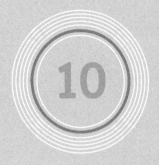

When it comes to dessert I am a purist. A craving for chocolate requires something with real chocolate or cocoa in it—carob just won't cut it, especially during pregnancy, when cravings come through loud and clear. You are either in the mood for a rich, delicious dessert (check out the Rich Chocolate Brownies on page 182), or you just want a sweet little nosh (like the Italian Lemon Cookies on page 179).

At first I planned to divide this chapter into two sections: the I-gotta-have-it traditional desserts (like the Ricotta Cheesecake on page 181) and the sounds-too-nutritional-to-be-yummy healthy desserts (like the Jam Dot Cookies on page 177). But it turns out that these categories are open to interpretation. If it does not have chocolate in it, it's not dessert to me, but our clients flip for Fruit Crisp (page 186). And I just love the Oatmeal Raisin Cookies with chocolate chips (page 176), but as far as my sister Gail is concerned, anything with sunflower seeds in it just cannot be called dessert. So here they all are in one batch for you to choose from. One thing you will not find are variations. Baking is more of a science than an art, so simply choose your favorite and channel your creativity into the toppings.

ABOUT SUGAR

One easy way to improve on the taste and quality of your baked goods (and coffee) is to use raw sugar, also known as evaporated cane sugar, instead of chemically processed granulated sugar.

For our Mothers & Menus baked goods, we use muscovado sugar, which is naturally processed from evaporated cane juice. Unlike most brown sugars, which are composed of refined white sugar with added molasses, muscovado is free from bleaching agents. It gets its name from the Spanish *muscabado*, which means "unrefined." Muscovado sugar is often found in health food stores or at Whole Foods Markets. Try to pick some up next time you go shopping and use it in place of dark brown sugar when you bake for a lighter, moister result.

Oatmeal Raisin Cookies • MAKES 4 DOZEN COOKIES

This is a new twist on an old-fashioned favorite, with shredded coconut and sunflower seeds pumping up the flavor, texture, and nutritional value. Your favorite chopped nuts can be used in addition to, or instead of, the seeds and coconut. Kids in the house (and the kid in you) will want to add in some chocolate chips or chunks.

    1 cup (2 sticks) unsalted butter, softened
    1½ cups packed dark brown sugar
    2 large eggs
    1 teaspoon pure vanilla extract
    1½ cups all-purpose flour
    1 teaspoon baking soda
    ½ teaspoon salt
    3 cups rolled oats
    1 cup raisins
    ½ cup sunflower seeds
    1 cup unsweetened dried coconut
    1 cup chopped nuts or bittersweet chocolate chips, or a combination, optional

Preheat the oven to 350°F.

With an electric mixer or working by hand with a wooden spoon, beat the butter and sugar together in a large bowl until light and fluffy. Add the eggs and vanilla and beat well.

In a small bowl, whisk together the flour, baking soda, and salt. Add to the butter mixture and mix until just combined. Stir in the oats, raisins, sunflower seeds, coconut, and nuts and/or chocolate chips if desired.

Drop the batter by rounded tablespoonfuls onto an ungreased cookie sheet about 2 inches apart. Bake until golden brown, 10 to 12 minutes. Cool for 1 minute and then transfer to a wire cooling rack to cool completely. Store in an airtight container for up to 1 week.

Express: I love this recipe because you can divide the batter into 4 logs and wrap and freeze them separately, pulling out a log whenever you have a craving. Bake straight from the freezer.

Jam Dot Cookies • MAKES ABOUT 20

These fabulous sugar-free cookies are naturally sweetened and contain no eggs or dairy, making them a delicious vegan option. Almonds are high in protein, magnesium, and vitamin E, and they beat out other nuts in fiber and calcium, giving this cookie high scores as a healthy, sweet treat! But don't tell that to your kids or your guests, who will delight in their chewy texture and rich flavor, enhanced with the sweet taste of preserves in every bite.

1 cup unblanched whole or sliced almonds
1 cup rolled oats
1 cup whole wheat flour
$\frac{1}{2}$ teaspoon ground cinnamon
  Pinch of salt
$\frac{1}{2}$ cup canola or another flavorless oil, such as safflower or sunflower
$\frac{1}{2}$ cup pure maple syrup
$\frac{1}{2}$ cup fruit-only preserves, preferably raspberry, strawberry, or apricot

Preheat the oven to 350°F. Lightly grease 2 cookie sheets or cover with parchment paper.

Combine the almonds, oats, flour, cinnamon, and salt in the bowl of a food processor and grind to a very fine meal. If any cakes on the bottom, just scrape it up with a spatula and pulse to reincorporate. Add the oil and maple syrup and pulse until combined into a uniform dough.

Roll the dough into 1-inch balls, and place 2 inches apart on the cookie sheets. Make an indentation in the center of each ball with your thumb or the back of a teaspoon. Bake until light golden brown, about 15 minutes. Remove from the oven and drop about 1 teaspoon of preserves into the center of each cookie. Bake for an additional 5 minutes to set. Transfer to a wire rack to cool completely. The cookies can be kept in an airtight tin in a cool, dry place for up to 1 week or in the freezer for up to 1 month. Be sure to pack the cookies with parchment or waxed paper or plastic wrap between layers so they don't stick to each other.

Two Lemon Cookies

When my daughter Nika, five, learned that I was writing a cookbook, she asked me (persistently) if I was going to include her recipe for Lemon Butter Cookies. "It is really easy, Mom. Just tell them to mix flour, eggs, milk, and lemon and put it in the oven and they'll have yummy cookies for their babies!"

Nika's recipe, which makes a classic, sweet, dense, American butter cookie, is great, but I was having a hard time deciding between it and one of Jen's favorites, an Italian cookie that is not too sweet, with a light, cakelike texture and a tangy lemon icing.

Of course, we had to conduct our own taste test, so I baked these with Nika and Sophie. They both pronounced the Lemon Butter Cookies to be their favorite, while I preferred the Italian ones myself. Here are both recipes so you and your family can decide for yourselves.

Lemon Butter Cookies • MAKES ABOUT 3 DOZEN COOKIES

3/4 cup (1½ sticks) unsalted butter, softened
1 cup sugar
1 large egg yolk
1 teaspoon pure vanilla extract
1 tablespoon grated lemon zest
¼ cup fresh lemon juice
1½ cups all-purpose flour
1½ teaspoons baking powder
½ teaspoon baking soda
Pinch of salt

With an electric mixer or working by hand with a wooden spoon, beat together the butter and sugar in a large bowl until light and fluffy. Add the yolk, vanilla extract, lemon zest and juice, and mix well. (The mixture may curdle because of the acidity in the lemon juice, but this is fine, it will come back together when you add the flour.)

In a small bowl, whisk together the flour, baking powder, baking soda, and salt. Mix into the butter mixture until just blended. Roll the dough into three logs 1 inch in diameter, wrap in plastic wrap, and refrigerate for at least 2 hours, or overnight (or freeze for up to 1 month).

Preheat the oven to 350°F.

Slice the dough into ¼-inch-thick slices. Place 2 inches apart on ungreased cookie sheets. Bake until light golden brown, 8 to 10 minutes (10 to 12 if baking straight from the freezer). Cool for 1 minute before removing to a wire rack to cool completely. Store in an airtight container in a cool, dry place for up to 1 week.

Italian Lemon Cookies • MAKES ABOUT 3 DOZEN COOKIES

½ cup (1 stick) unsalted butter, softened

½ cup sugar

3 large eggs

2 teaspoons grated lemon zest

2 cups all-purpose flour

2 teaspoons baking powder

Pinch of salt

Lemon Icing (recipe follows), optional

Preheat the oven to 350°F. Lightly grease a cookie sheet.

With an electric mixer or by hand with a wooden spoon, beat together the butter and sugar in a large bowl until light and fluffy. Add the eggs, one at a time, and mix until fully blended. Stir in the lemon zest.

In a medium bowl, whisk together the flour, baking powder, and salt. Add to the butter mixture, mixing until just blended. Using a mini ice cream scoop or 2 teaspoons, drop balls of dough, about 2 inches apart, onto the cookie sheet. Bake until lightly browned, 8 to 10 minutes. Transfer the cookies to a wire rack and let cool completely before icing.

Dip the cookies, upside down, into the icing, and allow them to set, right side up, on a wire rack before storing. Store in an airtight container in a cool, dry location for up to 1 week.

Lemon Icing • MAKES ABOUT ½ CUP

1 tablespoon unsalted butter, softened

1½ cups confectioner's sugar

½ teaspoon grated lemon zest, or more to taste

Juice of ½ lemon

In a small bowl, mix together the butter, sugar, lemon zest, and juice. If the icing is too thick, stir in 1 tablespoon of cold water.

Ultra-Energy Bar • MAKES 2 DOZEN BARS

There are so many energy bars available today, but making your own will take minutes of your time, reassure you that it's filled with only the best ingredients, and allow you to customize it exactly to your preferences. These bars freeze very well, so whip up a batch and wrap individually for a grab-and-go snack.

1 cup pure maple syrup
2/3 cup chunky natural peanut butter
2 2/3 cups rolled oats
1 cup whole wheat flour
1/4 cup soy protein powder or whey protein powder
1 teaspoon ground cinnamon
1/2 cup wheat germ
1/2 cup unsweetened dried coconut
1/2 cup raisins
1/2 cup chopped walnuts

Preheat the oven to 350°F. Lightly grease a 9 × 13-inch baking pan.

Use the back of a wooden spoon to mix the syrup and peanut butter together in a large bowl until well blended.

In a separate bowl, stir together the oats, flour, protein powder, cinnamon, wheat germ, coconut, raisins, and nuts. Mix into the peanut butter mixture to make a uniform dough. Press into the prepared pan. The mixture will be slightly sticky, but should still spread easily into the pan with greased fingers.

Bake until golden brown, about 25 minutes. Cut while warm into 1½ × 3-inch bars, and allow to cool completely in the pan. Wrap each bar individually and store in an airtight container for up to 1 week or freeze for up to 1 month.

Ricotta Cheesecake • MAKES ONE 10-INCH CAKE

This creamy yet light, citrus-flavored cheesecake will satisfy the strongest cravings for cheesecake, and it is unbelievably easy to prepare. It does need time to set, however, so you may want to make it a day ahead. Serve plain or with fresh berries.

1 tablespoon unsalted butter for the pan
1½ cups coarsely ground vanilla wafer cookies
3 pounds fresh ricotta cheese
1½ cups sugar
6 large eggs
1 teaspoon pure vanilla extract
1 teaspoon orange extract
Grated zest of 1 orange
½ cup fresh orange juice

Place a rack in the center of the oven. Preheat the oven to 325°F. Generously butter a 10-inch springform pan and coat with 1 cup of the cookie crumbs.

In a large bowl, whisk together the ricotta, sugar, eggs, vanilla and orange extracts, and orange zest and juice. Pour the batter into the pan and sprinkle the remaining ½ cup of cookie crumbs over the top. Bake until the cake jiggles only slightly at the center when the pan is tapped, about 1 hour.

Remove from the oven and let cool completely. Once cool, cover the pan tightly and refrigerate for at least 8 hours, or up to 3 days.

Release the sides of the pan and remove from the bottom. Cut the cake into slices and serve.

Rich Chocolate Brownies • MAKES 2 DOZEN BROWNIES

These brownies are all about the chocolate—the better the quality, the richer they will be. Using unsweetened dark chocolate means you'll be getting all of the health benefits of chocolate with less sugar and fat than milk chocolate. Be prepared for the intense flavor of these brownies, and consider cutting them into bite-size portions for a satiating, two-bite chocolate fix.

½ cup (1 stick) unsalted butter, plus extra for the pan
5 ounces best-quality unsweetened chocolate
1½ cups sugar
2 teaspoons pure vanilla extract
Pinch of salt
4 large eggs
1 cup all-purpose flour
1 cup chopped hazelnuts, pecans, almonds, or walnuts, optional

Preheat the oven to 350°F. Butter a 9 × 13-inch baking pan.

Melt the butter and chocolate together in a small saucepan over low heat. Transfer to a small bowl and set aside to cool completely. (This may take 15 to 20 minutes, but waiting it out makes a difference in the end result: warm chocolate can cook the eggs, giving you a cakelike finish, whereas a cool chocolate base will give you a truly fudgy brownie.)

Stir the sugar, vanilla, and salt into the chocolate. Add the eggs, one at a time, beating well each time using a wooden spoon.

Fold in the flour and nuts, if using. Mix just enough to blend thoroughly.

Spread out the batter (it will be very thick) in the pan evenly and bake until a toothpick inserted in the center comes out with moist crumbs clinging to it, 20 to 24 minutes.

Cool completely (or as long as you can hold out) and then cut into 24 pieces. If individually wrapped and stored in an airtight container, these brownies will keep well for up to 1 week, or they can be frozen for up to 1 month.

ABOUT CHOCOLATE

Chocolate's scientific name, *Theobroma cacao*, literally translates as "fruit of the gods." Of course, this doesn't mean that you should replace your fruit intake with chocolate, but rest assured that when you satiate that occasional craving with a small piece of good dark chocolate, you are actually doing your heart a favor. Like vitamins A, B_1, C, D, and E, chocolate has been found to increase good cholesterol levels (HDL) and contains flavonoids, which increase antioxidant levels in your body. But not all chocolate is created equal: the powerful flavonoids are found in the dark varieties of chocolate with a high percentage of cocoa (aim for 70 percent or more), and are stripped away in the process of creating milk chocolate. Do remember, however, that cocoa also contains caffeine, so bear that in mind when you choose to indulge (and enjoy your chocolate earlier in the day).

Devilicious Cupcakes • MAKES 1 DOZEN CUPCAKES OR 2 DOZEN MINICUPCAKES

These cupcakes come with a warning. Moist, sophisticated, and able to satisfy the deepest craving for chocolate, these could even convert a plain vanilla lover! Finish with Dark Chocolate Glaze (opposite) for a chocoholic frenzy.

　　1 cup boiling water
　　1 cup best-quality cocoa powder
　½ cup milk
1½ teaspoons pure vanilla extract
　　2 cups all-purpose flour
1¼ teaspoons baking soda
　½ teaspoon salt
　　1 cup (2 sticks) unsalted butter, softened
1¼ cups packed dark brown sugar
　¾ cup granulated sugar
　　4 large eggs

Preheat the oven to 350°F. Line a 12-slot muffin tin with paper liners and set aside.

In a small bowl, whisk together the water and cocoa until smooth. Stir in the milk and vanilla.

In a separate bowl, whisk together the flour, baking soda, and salt.

With an electric mixer or working by hand with a wooden spoon, beat the butter and brown and granulated sugars together in a large bowl until light and fluffy. Add the eggs, one at a time, beating well after each addition.

Add the flour mixture to the batter in thirds, alternating with the cocoa mixture, and starting and ending with the flour. Mix until smooth.

Scoop the batter into the muffins cups, filling them three-fourths full. Bake until a toothpick inserted in the center of a cupcake comes out clean, 22 to 25 minutes. Let cool for 10 minutes in the pan, then remove to a wire rack and cool completely. Store the cupcakes in an airtight container for up to 4 days or wrap individually and freeze for up to 1 month.

Dark Chocolate Glaze • MAKES 2 CUPS

The promise of this glaze relies heavily on its chocolate source, so invest in good stuff with at least 60 percent cocoa content, and you will be delighted with the results.

12 ounces best-quality bittersweet chocolate, coarsely chopped
6 tablespoons unsalted butter, cut into small pieces

Melt the chocolate with ¾ cup of cold water in a small saucepan over low heat until smooth. Remove from the heat and stir in the butter, 2 to 3 pieces at a time, and continue stirring until perfectly smooth. Let cool slightly, stirring occasionally, until the glaze reaches the desired consistency.

If the glaze becomes too thick, reheat it gently in a heat-proof bowl set over a pan of hot water, or in the microwave. It will keep refrigerated in an airtight container for up to 3 weeks.

Express: For a quick but impressive dessert, drizzle Dark Chocolate Glaze over any fresh fruit: baby bananas, berries of all kinds, oversized peaches, pears, or apricots. Sprinkle with dried coconut and garnish with fresh mint.

Fruit Crisp • MAKES ONE 10-INCH CRISP

This is a quick-and-easy dessert to make anytime, but it is especially nice when you find yourself with more fruit than you can eat, since it can be made with almost any seasonal fruit. Enjoy as is or pair it with a scoop of ice cream or some crème fraîche. Either way, this dessert is a big hit with children and adults alike.

1 cup plus 1 tablespoon all-purpose flour

1 cup packed dark brown sugar

2 teaspoons ground cinnamon

Pinch of salt

½ cup (1 stick) cold unsalted butter, cut into small pieces

1 cup rolled oats and/or ½ cup chopped nuts, optional

8 cups sliced fruit, such as apples, pears, peaches, or plums (about 2 pounds); or 8 cups berries, such as blueberries, blackberries, raspberries; or a combination

2 teaspoons fresh lemon juice

Preheat the oven to 375°F.

In a medium bowl, whisk together 1 cup of the flour, the sugar, 1 teaspoon of the cinnamon, and the salt until well blended. Use your fingertips or a pastry cutter to work in the butter (alternatively, you can pulse the mixture in a food processor), until the mixture resembles coarse meal. Add the oats and nuts, if desired, and set aside the topping.

Gently toss the fruit with the lemon juice, remaining teaspoon of cinnamon, and remaining tablespoon of flour in a 10-inch pie plate. Top with the crumble mixture and bake until the fruit is tender and bubbling around the edges and the topping is deep golden, about 40 minutes. Let cool at least slightly and serve warm or at room temperature.

Express: Make a big batch of topping and freeze in 2-cup containers for a fast, last-minute dessert. No need to defrost, simply pull from the freezer and use a fork to break up the crumble mixture before spreading over the filling.

Balsamic-Macerated Strawberries • SERVES 2

Quintessentially Italian, this simple dessert is stunning on its own, with Lemon Cookies (page 178), or spooned over pound cake. Buy organic summer berries for maximum flavor.

1 pint strawberries, hulled and sliced
¼ cup sugar
2 tablespoons balsamic vinegar
Mint sprigs for garnish

Put the berries in a small bowl and toss gently with the sugar. Cover and allow the berries to macerate, stirring occasionally, for at least 2 hours, or up to 8 hours in the refrigerator. A thick, ruby-red syrup will form as the berries sit.

When ready to serve, add the balsamic vinegar and stir.

Baked Apples with Nuts, Raisins, and Spices • SERVES 4

This warm, rich dessert is a great alternative to cookies and cakes, and makes a great comfort food. Dress apples up with whipped cream or down with a scoop of frozen yogurt. Although you can enjoy this treat year-round, it is especially fun to make in the fall and winter months, when apples are at their peak and the brisk air has us craving a warm dessert. This is great to make with children (see Real World, opposite), and everyone will enjoy the lingering aroma of nutmeg and cinnamon throughout your home.

4 large, firm, tart apples, such as Winesap, Granny Smith, or Jonagold
1 tablespoon fresh lemon juice
½ cup packed dark brown sugar or maple syrup
¼ cup golden raisins
⅓ cup pecans or walnuts, toasted (see page 70) and finely chopped
1 teaspoon ground cinnamon
¼ teaspoon ground nutmeg
4 teaspoons unsalted butter, cut into bits
½ cup apple cider or water

Preheat the oven to 350°F.

Core the apples, leaving them whole, or cut them in half and remove the cores with a small knife. Sprinkle with the lemon juice. Place in a glass or other nonreactive baking dish. (Put halved apples cored sides up.)

Mix together the sugar with the raisins, pecans, cinnamon, and nutmeg. Fill the apples or the centers of the apple halves with the mixture. You may find yourself with some mixture spilling over into the pan—this is fine and will be extra delicious when baked.

Dot the apples with butter and pour the apple cider into the bottom of the dish. Cover the dish with a lid or foil and bake for 25 minutes. Uncover and baste the apples with the juices from the pan. Bake until the apples feel tender when pierced with a knife, but not mushy, 10 to 15 minutes. Serve warm or at room temperature.

I made these apples with Rafael, two, as my assistant and Noah, six months, sitting in his high chair observing. It took 30 to 40 minutes to prep because we took our time: helping Rafael pour the ingredients into the bowl, pausing so he could taste the lemon, counting and recounting the apples, sampling the raisins, apple scrapings, and brown sugar (yum!).

I put them in the oven before serving dinner so they were done just in time for dessert. Mmm good—they turned out delicious!! We topped them with a no-sugar-added whole fruit peach sorbet. This made for a nice hot-cold contrast, which hit the spot. Rafael was so proud to serve it up to Daddy Gregory and everyone enjoyed the sweet treat.

Andrea Cordero Fage, New York, NY

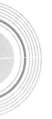

Poached Peaches with Raspberries and Whipped Cream · SERVES 4

During the summer, when peaches are fragrant and tinged with red, few desserts can rival a poached peach with raspberries and cream. Garnished with fresh mint, and served in a glass bowl or balloon wine goblet, these are spectacularly pretty. After serving the peaches, use the flavorful poaching syrup to sweeten home-made lemonade or herbal iced tea.

1½ cups sugar
½ vanilla bean, split lengthwise
　 Zest of 1 lemon or orange, removed
　　 with a vegetable peeler in strips
4 perfectly ripe peaches
　 Whipped Cream (recipe follows)
1 pint raspberries
4 sprigs fresh mint

Put the sugar in a medium saucepan, add 3 cups of cold water, and stir well to start dissolving the sugar. Add the vanilla bean and lemon zest and cook over medium-low heat until the sugar has completely dissolved, about 10 minutes.

Place the peaches in the syrup and cook over low heat until tender, 5 to 7 minutes, depending on their ripeness. Let the peaches cool in the syrup. Cover and refrigerate until chilled, several hours, or up to 2 days.

To serve, remove the peaches from the liquid, slip off their skins, and cut the fruits in half along their seams. Remove the pits and reassemble the peaches in 4 individual bowls. Top each with some whipped cream and raspberries, and garnish with mint. Drizzle a little of the poaching liquid over the top, if desired.

Whipped Cream • MAKES 1 CUP

　　1 cup heavy cream
　　2 tablespoons sugar
　　1 teaspoon pure vanilla extract

With an electric mixer or working by hand with a wire whisk, whip the cream until it starts to thicken. Add the sugar and vanilla and continue whipping until the cream forms soft peaks. If you would like to prepare the cream ahead of time, whip for slightly less time, and whip briefly just before serving.

ABOUT RASPBERRIES

Low in sugar, but high in vitamin C, potassium, and flavonoids, raspberries are clearly a terrific fruit to enjoy. But they are more multifaceted than they appear. In Chinese medicine, they are regarded as a tonic for the kidneys and liver, and are used to prevent anemia. In the tradition of magic, raspberries represent protection and love. They are served as a love-inducing food, and pregnant women carry their leaves to alleviate the discomforts of pregnancy and childbirth. Raspberry leaf tea is widely available as an infusion to support female reproductive systems. However, its effects on pregnant women have not yet been determined, so get clear on the facts prior to using.

11

Breakfasts

Still eschewing the most important meal of the day for a grande latte? Not for long. If you are lucky enough not to have morning sickness, then perhaps you are still getting away with starting your day without any food. As you grow bigger, though, so will your need for energy, and you will find (yet again) that Mom was right about the breakfast thing. (Just wait until you catch yourself giving your kids the most-important-meal spiel.) When you are up at night due to pregnancy or baby, 8:00 A.M. can feel like lunchtime, but psychologically, you are not ready for a soup and salad. The following breakfasts are laden with fuel to give you the energy to start (or continue) your day with a great kickoff.

If you do have morning sickness, start your day with a prebreakfast snack. Keep some easy-to-eat food by your bedside table, such as crackers or a banana— whatever you find works for you. My midwife's tip did wonders for me: I put a glass of ginger ale and a straw by my bed before going to sleep. When I woke up, I took a couple of sips through the straw before my feet hit the floor, so that by the time I made it to the kitchen, I had a little something inside of me. Also note that soon enough in addition to breakfast, you will probably need a midmorning snack, such as yogurt or nuts, to make it all the way to lunch.

Tomato, Herb, and Goat Cheese Frittata • SERVES 2

What I love about frittatas during pregnancy is that because they are not folded, you don't risk the chance that the eggs are not well done throughout. This particular recipe has me hooked. Not only is it easy to make and delicious to eat, it is also pleasing to the eye. When making it for my kids, I call it egg pizza and put on their favorite topping. This classic breakfast turns into a quick-and-easy lunch or dinner when filled out with a salad and crusty bread. It works well with whatever mixture of cheese and vegetables you have in the house. Try sautéed spinach, zucchini, or mushrooms instead of the tomato and replace the goat cheese with mozzarella, feta, or cheddar for some interesting alternatives.

Frittatas keep beautifully overnight in the fridge, so make the full recipe and save half for a meal the next day.

    5 large eggs
       Pinch of salt
 1½ teaspoons olive oil
    1 ripe plum tomato, seeded and chopped
    1 tablespoon mixed finely chopped herbs, such as chives,
          dill, parsley, tarragon, or basil; or 1 teaspoon dried
    2 tablespoons fresh goat cheese
       Freshly ground pepper

Preheat the oven to 450°F.

Beat the eggs in a small bowl with the salt. Heat the olive oil in a small ovenproof skillet over medium heat. Pour the eggs into the pan and let them sit undisturbed for about 10 seconds, so that the eggs begin to set. Then use a spatula to gently push the eggs toward the center of the pan, tilting the pan to allow uncooked eggs to run out underneath toward the edge of the pan.

When the eggs are semifirm, after 3 to 4 minutes, sprinkle the top with the tomato, herbs, and cheese. Transfer the pan to the oven, and bake until the frittata is puffy but not brown, about 4 minutes. Season with salt and pepper, cut into wedges, and serve.

FEELING GREEN: If you are having a hard time with eggs, a frittata may work well for you. Use a mild cheese such as mozzarella or cheddar, preferably grated, and spread over the top. Leave the eggs in the oven for 30 seconds longer to ensure they are cooked through.

FEELING FOOD: Top with a couple of slices of your favorite cheese before transferring to the oven. Once cooked, put on a plate and add slices of avocado for a creamy, cheesy, but healthy breakfast.

FEELING FULL: Use 3 egg whites and 2 whole eggs and reduce the goat cheese to 1 tablespoon to lighten things up. Do not go all white for two reasons—first, you will be missing out on all of the nutrients found in egg yolks, and second, the frittata will not come out quite as nicely.

REAL WORLD

My mother-in-law was coming over for lunch, so I decided to try out the frittata. I went out to get all of my ingredients (organic, of course!) and also bought a skillet that could be used on the stove and in the oven. I went with a goat cheese with herb and garlic, but because that was already salty, I did not salt the eggs (my doctor says I need to be extra careful about salt and high blood pressure since I am pregnant with twins). I used fresh dill and chives and, of course, the tomatoes. It was so fluffy and delicious. I loved how it made me look like such a great cook, even though I did it in no time. My husband, Lee, and his mom, Lillian, were so impressed. I plan to make this a staple of our weekends. I can already envision all the many other combinations I can make—with onions, asparagus, spinach—you name it!

Yael K. Hershfield, Palm Beach Gardens, FL

Granola Your Way • MAKES 6 CUPS

Many of our clients are addicted to our granola, which features whole grain oats, almonds, raisins, coconut, and sesame and sunflower seeds. The combo is lightly sweetened with maple syrup and enriched with wheat germ to make a power-packed breakfast, which can be served with milk or yogurt. It is also a great snack to nibble on its own. Customize this basic recipe to your taste: substitute pecans or walnuts for the almonds, chopped dried apricots or cherries for the raisins, and pumpkin seeds for the sunflower seeds, for example.

6 cups rolled oats
1 cup sliced almonds or other nuts
½ cup pure maple syrup
⅓ cup mild vegetable oil, such as safflower, canola, or sunflower
½ cup wheat germ
1 cup unsweetened dried coconut
1 cup hulled sunflower seeds
2 tablespoons sesame seeds
1 cup raisins or bite-size pieces of other dried fruit

Preheat the oven to 350°F.

Spread the oats and almonds on a large baking sheet. Toast in the oven, stirring often, until golden, 15 minutes.

Combine the maple syrup and oil in a small saucepan and bring to a boil. While the mixture is heating, add the wheat germ, coconut, and sunflower and sesame seeds to the oats and mix with a wooden spoon. Pour the maple syrup mixture over the oat mixture and mix well. Bake, stirring occasionally, until the granola is a rich golden brown, 10 minutes.

Let cool completely. Mix in the raisins and store in an airtight container for up to 5 days.

FEELING GREEN: Colonial-era folk remedies mention the use of cranberries to fight nausea. Add some dried cranberries to this crunchy mixture and enjoy on its own, without milk.

FEELING FOOD: Up the coconut by another ½ cup and add in ½ cup of bittersweet chocolate chips to turn this into a trail-mix–type of treat. Or prepare as is and make parfaits by layering the granola with yogurt and some fresh berries.

FEELING FULL: When you are feeling full, a little goes a long way. Make half of the recipe and store in an airtight container. Enjoy over plain yogurt or fresh fruit or both.

Quinoa and Amaranth Breakfast Porridge • MAKES 3 CUPS

Quinoa and amaranth, two giants of the grain universe, have been revered throughout history for their strength-giving properties. Rich in protein, iron, magnesium, and phosphorus, this hot breakfast cereal is excellent fuel. If you cannot find one of the two grains, substitute millet, which is also high in protein and minerals. Serve with your choice of milk—almond, rice, soy, or dairy—and your favorite toppings. Leftover cereal can be kept in the refrigerator and reheated on the stovetop with a little milk.

²/₃ cup quinoa
¹/₃ cup amaranth
Pinch of salt
Milk for serving
Dried fruit and/or nuts for serving
Ground cinnamon for garnish

Combine the quinoa, amaranth, and salt with 2 cups of cold water in a small saucepan. Bring to a boil, then cover and simmer until thickened and cooked through, 20 to 25 minutes.

Stir in milk to taste, top with fruit or nuts and a sprinkling of cinnamon, and serve immediately.

FEELING GREEN: Turn this into a savory porridge by stirring in 1 teaspoon of olive oil, a sprinkle of Parmesan cheese, and some salt and pepper before serving.

FEELING FOOD: Powerful grains may not seem appealing when you are looking for some comfort food. But *au contraire* with this porridge, which can be sweetened with a drizzle of maple syrup. Opt for nuts and fruit for a warm, syrupy, creamy, and crunchy treat.

FEELING FULL: If you are avoiding processed breakfast cereals, this porridge is an excellent alternative. Opt for skim milk, fresh berries, and raw nuts for maximum taste and nutrients.

Whole Grain Pancakes • SERVES 3 TO 4

Drop by our home on a Saturday morning, and you will probably find me making these delicious pancakes with the kids. They have grown so accustomed to this version that when they tried out some regular pancakes the other day, they pronounced them "too doughy." This proved to me that you really can acclimate your taste buds—and theirs— to healthier eating. If you do not already have one, I strongly recommend a griddle, which is larger than a skillet, so that you can whip up several platefuls in a flash and join your family for breakfast.

Enjoy these with real maple syrup, jam, or Balsamic-Macerated Strawberries (page 187).

> 1 cup all-purpose flour
> ½ cup whole grain flour, such as buckwheat, millet, or whole wheat
> 3 tablespoons ground flax seeds
> 2 teaspoons baking powder
> 1 teaspoon salt
> 1 tablespoon sugar
> 1 teaspoon ground cinnamon
> 2 cups skim milk
> 2 large eggs
> Butter or oil for the pan

Whisk together the all-purpose and whole grain flours, flax seeds, baking powder, salt, sugar, and cinnamon in a large bowl.

Pour the milk into a medium bowl, add the eggs, and whisk until smooth. Stir the wet ingredients into the dry ingredients with a rubber spatula. Do not overmix: you should end up with a batter that is a little lumpy.

Heat a griddle or large skillet over medium-high heat and grease lightly with butter. Using a ⅓ cup measuring cup, drop the batter onto the pan, leaving room for the pancakes to spread. Wait until you see bubbles forming on the tops of the pancakes, 2 to 3 minutes, then flip, and cook until the bottoms are brown, another minute or so. Repeat with the remaining batter.

FEELING GREEN: These pancakes are a huge favorite with my feeling green moms because they are moist, without being greasy. Tuck a couple in a resealable plastic bag and carry them with you for a quick bite when you need to munch.

FEELING FOOD: Reduce the milk to 1¼ cups and stir in 4 tablespoons of melted butter. You will find these pancakes to be a little fluffier, while still packed with protein and omega-3. Of course, if that still feels too healthy, you can always mix in some chocolate chips.

FEELING FULL: Reverse the flour quantities—use 1 cup of whole grain and ½ cup of all-purpose—for a healthier version. Substitute high-sugar maple syrup with natural fruit syrup: Put a 10-ounce bag of frozen berries and 2 tablespoons of water in a small saucepan. Heat over medium-high heat, stirring occasionally, for about 5 minutes. Reduce the heat and simmer until the berries are softened, about 3 minutes.

ABOUT COOKING WITH KIDS

Bringing your children into the kitchen with you at a young age (about nine months) is a great way to spend quality time with them and get them to try out new foods. Preparing breakfast foods on the weekends is one way to go, when you don't have a hungry family waiting for their dinner. Although sometimes this works well at dinnertime—having the kids participate in the preparation can stall their cries for "Is dinner ready yet?" In our New York City apartment, there isn't room for all of us to comfortably (and safely) cook in the kitchen, so we sit around the breakfast table, and I pass the mixing bowl around for everyone to take a turn: Nika adds the flour, Ethan shakes the cinnamon, Sophie pours the milk and cracks the eggs. The end result isn't always perfect, and there is always much cleaning to be done. But the mess decreases as they grow, their love for cooking intensifies, and the time we spend together is priceless.

French Toast · SERVES 3 TO 4

This now classic American breakfast favorite originated in France, where it is called pain perdu, *literally, "lost bread." Lost in cream, eggs, and butter, that is. This recipe respects the classic, without completely submitting to it, by calling for milk rather than cream. While admittedly basic, it can be tweaked in a number of ways to make it healthier or richer. See the Feeling . . . variations for some ideas.*

1 cup milk
4 large eggs
1 teaspoon pure vanilla extract
6 thick slices brioche or challah bread
3 tablespoons unsalted butter
   Maple syrup, honey, or jam for serving

Whisk the milk, eggs, and vanilla together in a shallow baking dish. Add the bread slices, one at a time, turning in the mixture until saturated.

Melt the butter in a griddle or skillet over medium heat. Add as many slices of bread as will comfortably fit in one layer. Cook until the bottoms are golden brown, 2 to 3 minutes, then flip and cook, until the second sides are a rich golden color, 1 to 2 minutes. Repeat with the remaining slices of bread.

Serve topped with maple syrup.

FEELING GREEN: Replace the brioche or challah bread with thinly sliced sandwich bread, such as a whole wheat or white, which will have a firmer texture than the custardy egg breads. Dip lightly to coat, but do not saturate the toast, so the bread will not be too soggy and rich for your palate.

FEELING FOOD: Take these to the next level by following the egg dip with a dip in shredded coconut or finely chopped nuts—such as pistachios or almonds—in a shallow bowl. Top with orange marmalade, sautéed bananas, or cinnamon sugar.

FEELING FULL: Use skim, rice, soy, or almond milk. Add 1 teaspoon of ground cinnamon to the egg mixture. Use 6 thin slices of whole grain bread. Top with fresh fruit for a beautiful finish to your healthy breakfast.

REAL WORLD

Just this morning we made the Feeling Full version with great results. First, my husband, Adam, took Siena, four and a half, and Cira, twenty-two months, to the Telluride farmers market to buy organic eggs and summer cherries to enjoy with the toast. The owners of the White Buffalo Farm said they acquired their cherry trees from an estate that once produced cherries for several presidents (these cherries certainly made us proud to be Americans!). Upon their return, Siena helped break the eggs and stir the batter while sitting atop the counter, and I hoisted Cira high on my hip to see the griddle action. The kids really loved cooking with me and were very proud of the delicious result, which we all enjoyed tremendously.

Taunya van der Steen, Aspen, CO

Ultimate Bran Muffins • MAKES 1 DOZEN MUFFINS

We do not take the word "ultimate" lightly. This muffin really deserves the title. Packed with fiber and additional iron from the molasses and raisins, it lives up to the beneficial properties associated with bran muffins. But its rich flavor and moist and chewy texture make it a delicious crowd-pleaser as well. Do not let the long ingredient list fool you—this batter will be ready in three simple steps. Look for unprocessed miller's bran in your local health food store or Whole Foods Market.

1¼ cups all-purpose flour
1½ teapoons baking soda
1½ teaspoons baking powder
1 teaspoon ground cinnamon
Pinch of salt
1 cup unprocessed miller's bran
1 cup buttermilk, or milk
2 large eggs
⅓ cup mild vegetable oil, such as safflower, canola, or sunflower
¼ cup molasses
⅓ cup packed dark brown sugar
½ teaspoon pure vanilla extract
½ cup golden raisins
½ cup dark raisins

Preheat the oven to 400°F. Line a 12-slot muffin tin with paper liners.

In a medium bowl, whisk together the flour, baking soda, baking powder, cinnamon, and salt. Set aside.

In a large bowl, mix the bran with the buttermilk, eggs, oil, molasses, sugar, vanilla, and raisins, and allow to sit for 10 minutes to soften the bran.

Add the flour mixture all at once to the bran mixture and mix rapidly until just blended. Scoop the batter into the muffin cups, filling them nearly to the top. Bake until a toothpick inserted in the center of a muffin comes out clean, 18 to 20 minutes.

Remove the muffins from the tin and cool completely on a wire rack. The muffins are best the day they are made, but can be frozen for up to 2 weeks.

FEELING GREEN: Ginger is known for relieving nausea and works very well in this recipe. Add 2 tablespoons of ground ginger to the bran mixture. For a drier snack, consider omitting the raisins.

FEELING FOOD: Enjoy these warm out of the oven with just a smidgeon of butter melted into them. Yummy!

FEELING FULL: Replace the all-purpose flour with whole wheat flour and add 2 tablespoons of flax seeds to the flour mixture. Reduce the vegetable oil to ¼ cup. When mixing the wet ingredients, add ½ cup unsweetened applesauce and 1 cup of shredded carrots. Omit the molasses. The result is still delicious but has even more protein and iron (if possible!).

REAL WORLD

Like most children, my two-year-old son, Jamie, is a big fan of anything vaguely resembling a cake, but I was uncertain if bran muffins would be too healthy and not enough of a sweet. I needn't have worried, as he gave these a big thumbs-up. I made minor changes to the ingredients listed, using half white and half whole wheat flour, and maple syrup instead of molasses, which I couldn't get ahold of. I also substituted cut-up dried apricots for half the raisins for additional flavor. Being in my third trimester, I am particularly concerned about my nutritional intake. The great thing about these muffins is that they totally hit the spot when you're craving something sweet, but have the added value of being packed with protein and iron.

The batter is incredibly easy and child-friendly to make, though honestly my son was more interested in ensuring that the muffins would be done in time for his dessert than actually mixing the ingredients. When the muffins were ready, he ate three small "cakies" as fast as he could fit them in his mouth! My husband Lior's eyes lit up when he ate his one—which also turned into three—and I know that this will be a strong breakfast favorite with him, too.

Abigail Levy-Gurwitz, London, England

Lemon-Blueberry Corn Muffins • MAKES 1 DOZEN MUFFINS

These muffins are a big hit with my family. My kids love how delicious they are, I love how effortless they are to make, and we all love the smell in the house while they are baking. The cornmeal adds a whole grain goodness, sweetness, and color to these muffins. Although these muffins are a summer favorite with fresh berries, you may find yourself making them at other times of the year with frozen berries. Add frozen blueberries straight from the freezer, and at the last second; otherwise they turn the batter greenish-blue.

1½ cups all-purpose flour
½ cup yellow cornmeal
2 teaspoons baking powder
½ teaspoon salt
½ cup (1 stick) unsalted butter, melted and cooled
¾ cup sugar
2 large eggs
1 cup milk
Grated zest of 1 lemon
1½ cups fresh blueberries, or 1 (10-ounce) bag frozen blueberries

Preheat the oven to 400°F. Line a 12-slot muffin tin with paper liners.

In a large bowl, whisk together the flour, cornmeal, baking powder, and salt. In a separate bowl, whisk together the butter, sugar, eggs, milk, and zest. Pour over the flour mixture and mix together with a few light strokes. Fold in the berries. Do not overmix; this batter will not be completely smooth.

Divide the batter among the muffin cups, filling them about three-quarters full. Bake until a toothpick inserted in the center of a muffin comes out clean, about 15 minutes.

Remove the muffins from the tin and cool completely on a wire rack. The muffins should be eaten within 1 day (and probably will be!).

FEELING GREEN: Prior to folding in the berries, fill 6 muffin cups with the lemon-cornmeal batter. Then fold in ¾ cup of berries and pour the batter into the remaining 6 cups. Enjoy the plain ones and save the fruit ones for the rest of your family.

FEELING FOOD: Pair warm muffins with Honey-Orange Cream Cheese (recipe follows).

FEELING FULL: Replace the butter with ½ cup of unsweetened applesauce. Reduce the sugar to ¼ cup and use skim milk. Up the berries to 2 cups for added natural sweetness.

Honey-Orange Cream Cheese • MAKES ABOUT 1 CUP

In exactly 2 minutes you can take cream cheese to a new level when you prepare this fragrant, and not too sweet, spread. This is a great way to impress with ease at a weekend brunch or on a picnic.

1 (8-ounce) package cream cheese, softened
    Grated zest of 1 orange
2 tablespoons honey

Mix all the ingredients until well blended. Store in an airtight container for up to 1 week.

REAL WORLD

I made these this morning with my daughter, Lucy. At twenty-two months, she is already a pro at muffin making, with her own style and preferences. First she dumped everything in, and then she mixed everything with a very small teaspoon, definitely going beyond the "few light strokes" called for in the recipe. Lucy scooped the batter and filled many of the minimuffin cups herself—although it wasn't the only place the batter landed.

Lucy ate a whole one as soon as it cooled and pronounced it "'licious." Brian, my husband, agreed. I loved them for a few reasons: Normally I am a big fan of corn muffins, but sometimes find them to be too cakelike. This one had the cornmeal taste that I enjoy, but, surprisingly, was not too sweet. I also loved how the berries kept their shape. Often they will disappear into the batter, but these were still whole.

Laurie Berkner, New York, NY

Date Nut Bread · MAKES TWO 8-INCH LOAVES

Dark, moist, and loaded with dates and nuts, this rich and filling bread tastes more like a cake. Wrap and freeze a loaf for up to 1 month. Defrost it on the countertop; it should be ready to enjoy within 1½ hours.

Organic Medjool dates may be harder to find than standard supermarket ones and are quite pricey, but their buttery flavor and smooth texture are a great addition to the recipe. Enjoy any leftover dates when you crave something sweet. Or tuck a walnut into each one for a Moroccan-style dessert. If you are out of nutmeg, ginger, or cloves, replace them all with 1 teaspoon of allspice.

1 cup all-purpose flour

1 cup whole wheat flour

1 teaspoon baking powder

¾ teaspoon baking soda

¼ teaspoon salt

1 teaspoon ground cinnamon

½ teaspoon ground nutmeg

½ teaspoon peeled and grated fresh ginger

½ teaspoon ground cloves

½ cup (1 stick) unsalted butter, softened

⅔ cup packed dark brown sugar

2 large eggs

2 very ripe bananas, cut into small chunks

1 cup unsweetened applesauce

1½ cups chopped dates, preferably organic Medjool

1 cup chopped walnuts

Preheat the oven to 350°F. Grease two 8 × 4-inch loaf pans.

In a medium bowl, whisk together the all-purpose and whole wheat flours, baking powder, baking soda, salt, cinnamon, nutmeg, ginger, and cloves. Set aside.

With an electric mixer or working by hand with a wooden spoon, beat the butter and sugar in a large bowl until fluffy and light in color. Add the eggs, one at a time, and beat until smooth. Add the bananas and mix until well incorporated. Stir in the applesauce.

Add the flour mixture, dates, and walnuts to the wet ingredients and fold in until just blended. Divide the batter between the 2 pans and bake until a toothpick inserted in the center of each loaf comes out clean, 40 to 45 minutes. Cool for 10 minutes before removing from the pans. Let cool completely on a wire rack before slicing.

FEELING GREEN: Add an additional teaspoon of ginger to the flour mixture. After slicing the bread, toast and enjoy a drier, crispier version of this moist bread as an alternative to the plain toast and crackers you may be relying on.

FEELING FOOD: Toast the bread lightly and spread with Honey-Orange Cream Cheese (page 205).

FEELING FULL: Omit the butter, increase the applesauce to 2 cups, and decrease the sugar to $\frac{1}{3}$ cup for a tasty yet lighter result.

LEGEND HAS IT . . .

In biblical times, women used dates to activate delivery, help with recovery, and activate milk production. Later on, they mixed dates with milk and cinnamon to create an aphrodisiac and stimulate sexual desire (leading them to need still more dates, I imagine).

Breakfast Smoothies • SERVES 1

Smoothies are a quick-and-easy way to get the nutrients you need at the start of your day, as a snack, or for dessert. Incorporating one smoothie a day into your routine can help you get in your omega-3s, calcium or fruit, and some protein. And they always feel like a treat. This is also a great way to get children into the kitchen and nourish them in a fun and delicious way.

For each of the following flavors, combine all of the ingredients in a blender and blend on high speed until creamy.

Vanilla Nut

1 banana
1 tablespoon almond butter
½ teaspoon pure vanilla extract
¼ cup vanilla protein powder (see page 214)
1 cup cold almond, soy, rice, or dairy milk
1 tablespoon flax seed oil
4 ice cubes

Creamy Orange

1 cup fresh orange juice
½ cup vanilla yogurt
¼ cup vanilla protein powder (see page 214)
1 tablespoon flax seed oil
4 ice cubes

Very Berry

1 cup mixed fresh or frozen berries
½ cup vanilla yogurt
¼ cup vanilla protein powder (see page 214)
½ cup milk
1 tablespoon flax seed oil
4 ice cubes

FEELING GREEN: The Vanilla Nut might be your best bet, with its tasty but neutral flavors. Sip it slowly throughout the morning. If you need a tart treat, try the Very Berry.

FEELING FOOD: The Creamy Orange may remind you of the Creamsicles of your childhood. Or turn the Vanilla Nut into a chocolate–peanut butter smoothie by replacing the vanilla with chocolate protein powder.

FEELING FULL: The Very Berry is high in antioxidants, but you can fortify it further by dropping the yogurt and milk in favor of $\frac{1}{3}$ cup of unsweetened cranberry juice and $\frac{2}{3}$ cup of water. If this proves too tart for you, try adding 1 teaspoon of maple syrup or a sweetener of your choice.

REAL WORLD

With the berries so fresh and beautiful this summer, choosing a shake was easy. We went to the fruit stand and picked an assortment of strawberries, blueberries, and blackberries. Lee, five, and Maya, three, helped with measuring. The fun part was mixing it in the blender. To our surprise we ended up with a beautiful, bright purple color. My husband, Mike, and I loved it, as did Maya—she's my fruity one. Lee enjoyed making it, but did not want to taste it. All told, I was happy with the antioxidants we got, and even happier about the time we spent together.

Lola Scheiner, New York, NY

Creating the First Six Weeks

When my firstborn, Nika, arrived, I was in heaven.
I was so moved by the miracle of her perfection
and the birth experience that I did not notice how
tired I was. When I was checking out of the hospital,
a nurse looked over with great concern in her
eyes and asked me if I had any help.

"Help?" I asked.

"Yes," she said. "Help. You know, your mom, a friend, is someone going to be helping you when you get home?"

I thought to myself, No, I don't need that kind of help. I am a multitasker, a hard worker, a nurturer by nature. I don't need any help because I am actually going on vacation now from my working life, to be a mom to my baby.

I smiled at her and walked away, anxious to get home with my precious bundle.

It took a few weeks for her words to sink in. I held Nika all the time. I refused to buy a stroller because I did not want to put her down. I went out on walks every day and carried her on me wherever I went. I knew I was tired, but I thought that it was natural; eventually Nika would start sleeping and so would I.

The realization that I was exhausted came slowly, in the form of arguments with Dori and my mom, a first-time grandmother eager to help. They urged me to supplement with formula so they could take over some of the feedings, and I could get some sleep. I felt betrayed that they were not supporting me in my attempts to nurse. I was getting depleted, and my milk production was running low in the late evenings. I needed to eat more, drink more, and rest more, but for some reason, I couldn't find the time to do all three.

When Nika was four weeks old, I put her down for a nap and debated between taking a shower, eating something, or passing out. I opted for the shower and thought about what I could do to make my life a little easier. I had asked my housekeeper to come twice a week so the apartment was clean and the laundry was done. I thought that if I could get a handle on the food part, that would take a load off my shoulders. By the time Sophie was born, seventeen months later, I had spoken to enough moms to know that they, too, realized the need for additional support. I set up the company that would become Mothers & Menus, taking the quiet, peaceful Sophie along with me to my meetings. As Sophie turned two and a half, Ethan came along, grinning his way into our (previously) princess-filled home. Ethan was much needier than the girls had been, nursing every hour and a half, and constantly wanting to be held. But now I had the service I had dreamed of, as well as experience and the knowledge that eventually everything passes. I ate well, rested often, and found myself with an abundance of energy to be with my newborn, my girls, and my husband and could still make a little time for myself.

Getting to this place took me three children and four years, and I wanted to tell expectant, first-time moms all of the things that I wished someone had told me. It is a fine line to walk. On the one hand, I don't want to scare anyone; on the other hand, armed with the right information, people could be having babies in a completely different setting. Unlike Eastern cultures, where new parents are surrounded by close communities of supportive friends and family, our Western world has many of us living miles away from our support networks, with completely different demands on our lives.

I believe that when you have structures in place, you can tune into your inner parenting guide. It's not about what you can do—you just had a baby, you can do anything. It is about moving beyond survival mode, to creating: being conscious of your time and allocating it to your highest priorities—bonding with your baby, connecting with your spouse, getting rest, and eating well. If you take care of yourself, you can take better care of your baby. This chapter is about just one piece of the puzzle, but it's a big one and will affect your entire family in a positive way. Creating a food structure during pregnancy will provide you with some support, so you can tune into your baby's rhythm (instead of your hunger pains) and discover yourself as a mom. But these are also great staples to have when you are a not-so-new mom and need a fallback plan for quick snacks or meals. This is not a shopping list for the recipes provided, or even a comprehensive pantry list, but rather a list of shortcuts when you need to pull something together in the blink of an eye. Have these on hand for the first six weeks, and you will never go hungry.

Pantry

BEANS: Canned, please; now is not the time to soak. Canned beans are as nutritious as fresh ones, just make sure to rinse them well to remove excess sodium. For those who feel bloated after eating beans, look for smaller legumes, such as adzuki beans, lentils, split peas, and small white beans, which will be less prone to cause gas. Add a little vinaigrette to beans, and you have a protein-packed instant meal.

CHOCOLATE: Finally, traditional medicine has proven what I have known all along: chocolate doesn't just make you feel good, it is good for you! (Okay, so I *wished* it more than *knew* it.) Something about releasing the feel-good dopamine and providing antioxidant flavonoids—how much more do you really need to know? What you want is a real, cocoa-based chocolate (not milk chocolate) with a high percentage of cocoa (aim for 70 percent or more) and limited sugar content.

DRIED FRUIT: True, it is full of sugar (the natural kind), but it is also filled with fiber and iron and makes a healthful, always-ready snack or dessert when you want something sweet. Dried fruit can enhance a salad, give a lift to steamed rice, and is a delicious add-in to your morning porridge or cereal. Think figs, raisins, apricots, dates, shredded coconut, apple, mango, or pineapple chunks. You can find almost any fruit in its unsweetened, dried version, and a little goes a long way.

OATMEAL: Instant, of course. But please, make sure its sole ingredient is oats. I love the 100% Natural Whole Grain Instant Oatmeal by Old Wessex. Every morning, I cut up some fruit as I boil water for my coffee and the kids' oatmeal. Within minutes we are all sitting down for breakfast together. With fiber, iron, and protein in every serving, not to mention warmth and texture, oatmeal makes a great start to the day. And there is so much you can dress it up with—berries, apples and cinnamon, maple syrup, and walnuts. Look at all of the commercial brands with loads of add-in ingredients for inspiration and then create your own natural version.

DRIED PASTA: There comes a time when spaghetti and sauce just have to do for dinner. Look for whole wheat pasta or try some alternative pastas, such as quinoa or Jerusalem artichoke. Balance out your meal by adding some vegetables, preferably spinach or kale (when in a real rush I throw the frozen, chopped versions into the pasta water when the pasta is nearly done). Top off the pasta with some grated Parmesan for a fully nurturing and nourishing meal.

TOMATO SAUCE: There are many quality brands available; find the one that works for you. Look for one that does not overdo the sodium or the sugar and avoid ones with corn syrup.

PROTEIN POWDER: Often when we are tired, we will reach for a processed carbohydrate before fresh fruit, vegetables, or protein. Adding some whey or soy protein powder to your diet will not change that, but it will make it easier for you to balance things. I use chocolate powder to satisfy my cravings and blend it with some skim milk and ice along with a tablespoon of flax seed oil. Pick a flavor that you love and put a Post-it with instructions on the blender so any visitor can whip up a protein shake for you and join you for a quick and healthy treat. Look for some other suggestions for smoothies on page 208. You can find protein powders at health food stores or Whole Foods Markets.

Freezer

PREPARED FOOD: The best time to prepare food for yourself is before the baby arrives, while you still have time. When you are making your favorite soup or casserole, double up and freeze the rest in single-size portions, so you can defrost a meal easily. When your friends ask how they can help, tell them they can cook something for your freezer. Make sure to label everything clearly along with a "by when" date so you know when it is time to use it up. After that, either toss it out or pass it off to your husband if he is, like mine, very confident about (and proud of) his strong stomach.

FROZEN FRUIT: Think berries, peaches, mangos, or any mixed fruits that you can buy precut. Of course, fresh should be part of your diet, too, but stocking frozen fruit means you always have some sort of fruit on hand. Puree in a blender with plain yogurt or milk for a quick shake. Do not forget your flax seed oil and protein powder, but skip the ice, since the fruits are frosty enough. Toss frozen fruit into your oatmeal or defrost and use to top frozen waffles for some added sweetness along with vitamins and nutrients.

FROZEN VEGETABLES: You know you need to eat your vegetables, but they take so long to prepare! Hence the frozen vegetable, in all of its glorious, prewashed, precut, or prechopped glory, is a staple in our home. Starting with broccoli, and moving on to spinach, kale, green beans, and that carrot, corn, and pea mix kids adore is simply the easiest way to go when you do not have time to shop for or prepare fresh.

WAFFLES: At this point you may be thinking, Are you kidding me? Frozen waffles? In a cookbook with fabulous recipes for French Toast (page 200) and Whole Grain Pancakes (page 198)? But let me remind you that this chapter is all about taking the easy way out and making compromises. Taking shortcuts when needed will allow you to nourish yourself while managing everything else you have going on, whether it is morning sickness, a newborn, or a family of four. And if a couple of frozen whole grain waffles will help you get your morning started, then I am for them by all means. Of course, I recommend looking at the ingredients lists when buying waffles: look for ones made with whole grains, that are minimally sweetened, and, as always, the fewer the ingredients the better. Then pop them in the toaster and grab some fruit and a glass of skim milk, and voilà, you have just created a nourishing breakfast.

Refrigerator

MISO PASTE: Miso is a terrific food to eat anytime because it is rich in calcium and iron, but it is even more beneficial during pregnancy and nursing because it contains enzymes that aid in digestion. My husband, Dori, loves miso because it makes for such an easy snack. He just adds hot water, some optional cut-up scallion and tofu chunks, and he's got soup. For a richer version with variations, see page 58. You can buy miso in the Asian section of many supermarkets or at any health food store (look for it in the refrigerated section).

OILS: Wait—oils in the fridge? you ask. Yes. Oils such as flax seed oil, fish oil, and others that are sensitive to heat should be kept refrigerated. Even our old friend extra-virgin olive oil is best kept in the refrigerator so it does not become rancid. (When it does go bad, you will not be able to taste the difference, but your body will know it, because the great properties of the oils will be compromised.) But let's get back to the first oils I mentioned (flax and fish oil)—these are the oils with the famous omega-3, which you have heard about time and time again (see page 24). A simple way of incorporating these into your diet is by having them available and simply adding them to whatever you are having—some oil in your smoothie, on your salad (use a lot of lemon at first, until you get used to the taste), or drizzled over pasta.

NUTS: Wait—nuts in the fridge? You are having a déjà vu. Basically, nuts need to be refrigerated for the same reason oils do: the fat in the nuts is sensitive to heat and can go bad. This is why we generally recommend enjoying your nuts raw rather than roasted. Besides being higher in nutrients by retaining their vitamin B$_1$ (thiamine) properties, they are also easier to digest. Look to almonds, walnuts, pistachios, pecans, and cashews for some great fat, fiber, protein, other nutrients, and taste. Walnuts are particularly high in omega-3 and almonds contain the most calcium and fiber. But mix them up for variety and balance. Also, try some seeds like pine nuts, sunflower seeds, and pumpkin seeds for extra fat and crunch in your salads, pilafs, and snacks. Or simply grab a handful of nuts to tide you over until mealtime.

NUT BUTTER: So now you are catching my drift—oils and nuts should be refrigerated. When I say nut butter, most people think peanut butter, which is certainly a great, high-protein snack. However, some people avoid all peanuts during pregnancy and nursing. Explore the world of available nut butters, from almond to cashew. Your local health food store might be your best bet. Look for a nut butter that is made with raw nuts, not roasted, so that you can get the optimum nutrients out of it. If you are going to go roasted, however, just make sure that partially hydrogenated vegetable oils are not on the list of ingredients. You can even make nut butters at home if you are so inclined: put the nuts in a food processor, process away, and there you have it, nut butter. Top your morning toast or waffle with some nut butter and fruit—or eat it with a teaspoon out of the jar. My favorite treat when I was pregnant with Nika was a spoonful of nut butter pressed into some unsweetened chocolate chips—my take on a Reese's peanut butter cup.

SAUERKRAUT: Okay, I know, it looks a little funny on this bare bones survival list. But organic sauerkraut is one of our favorite foods for many reasons. Because of the natural fermentation that occurs when the cabbage is cultured, it creates the popular good-for-you bacteria acidophilus, which enhances digestion. Sauerkraut is supposed to help pregnant women with morning sickness. (I admit, I never tried this— if you do, please write me and tell me if it works!) Sauerkraut is supposed to be great for nursing colicky babies, helping them with digestion (again, I have not checked this theory out personally). But in our house, sauerkraut is just a snack that we love to eat—even more so knowing that it is good for us. Even my picky eater, Sophie, now four, loves it. So, if you like the taste of it, keep it in your fridge. But remember to look for organic sauerkraut that has been fermented while raw, not cooked, thereby allowing the fermentation process to take place naturally.

Weekly Groceries

With your pantry and freezer stocked, you need to have some food in your fridge on a weekly basis. One system I find to be most helpful is to make a list of everything we like to have and post it on the fridge. Include brand names, sizes, flavors—every detail—so family and friends can pitch in with the shopping and get you exactly what you want. It can be frustrating to open the fridge and find a six-pack of blueberry yogurt when all you want is plain (or vice versa). A detailed list also makes it easier for whoever is buying to get back to you as soon as possible (don't underestimate the importance of that) and avoid calling you twelve times (waking up the baby who just fell asleep) with the inevitable questions: "When you said low-fat did you mean skim or 1 percent?" "Was that enriched skim or regular?" "You sure you don't want chocolate milk?" I know that many husbands appreciate the list because it allows them to be helpful without having to bug you or forget anything. In fact, you'll appreciate having this list during those forgetful days of pregnancy. Better yet, if you have access to a supermarket delivery service, create a regular list and have them redeliver it every time you call in. Once again, the idea is to have you thinking as little as possible about anything other than you and your baby (and, trust me, your husband will enjoy the benefits of a relaxed mom and a full fridge).

Some of the things to remember for your list:

DAIRY: Write down your favorite milk, cheese, and yogurt. We love Stonyfield Farms Squeezers and plain yogurt. Freeze some for a healthy frozen yogurt treat.

EGGS: One trick I use is to boil a dozen eggs while I put away the groceries. This way, there is a quick protein snack ready whenever you need it.

FRUITS: Any fresh, seasonal fruit will do. Try and wash them and get them in a bowl—in the fridge or on your counter—as soon as you get home. A bag of even the most beautiful peaches that is shoved into a fruit drawer may stay there, forgotten, whereas a beautiful bowl filled with colorful treats will entice you to eat them more often.

VEGETABLES: I worked in technology for many years and was thrilled to try out many gadgets before their time. But my favorite technology of all—okay, other than my Blackberry, or my Tivo—is the one that allows farmers to prewash and precut vegetables and put them in a bag, which goes straight to my table. Mesclun greens, shredded cabbage, baby spinach, shredded carrots, you name it, I will buy it—not only because of the time I will save by getting lunch or dinner on the table faster, but also because of the increased likelihood that we will be eating those items since I will not have to deal with the prep work. The other way to pump up your vegetable intake is to go small: baby carrots and grape tomatoes are perfect things to pop in your mouth when you can't find time to make a proper meal, or while you are standing at the fridge, waiting for your inspiration for dinner to overtake you. If you have young children, put these veggies on a lower shelf so it is the first thing they see when they open the fridge.

And Finally

Whether or not you are a nursing mom, you need to drink a lot of water to keep up your energy and help out your body. But if you are nursing, this goes double for you, so buy cases of twenty-four half-liter bottles and distribute them throughout the house, wherever you usually find yourself sitting down. When you see one—drink! Make sure someone keeps replacing the empties or refills them with filtered tap water.

Acknowledgments

It took many "chefs" to cook up this book. The two who ladled up a generous serving of faith, patience, and hand-holding were Rica Allannic, my knowledgeable, warm editor, whose sharp and witty remarks made a first-time editorial process fun, and Kirsten Manges, my incredible agent, whose intelligent insight and uncanny ability to make the most honest comments in the nicest manner carried me through from the beginning to present day. I thank you both for believing in me and giving me this amazing opportunity. And to the supporting team at Clarkson Potter: Danielle Deschenes, Sydney Webber, Andrew Stanley, Jean McCall, Alice Peisch, Ann Gregory, and Kathleen Fleury—thank you so much for your contributions.

To the many wise women who have guided me throughout the years: Christine Thomas, Denise Spatafora, Gail Turel, Galia Granot, Jan Shapiro, Laura Rabhan, Lilly Berelovich, Lynn Kreaden, Marie Lumholtz, Sandra Fathi, and Sylvie Tendler, thank you for your unique and valuable support.

I have much gratitude for the mothers we serve at Mothers & Menus, including those who inspired the birth of this book and those who took time to contribute to it (and also those who tried and just couldn't make it in time). And for the talented team at Mothers & Menus whose dedication makes it all run so smoothly, especially Katie Haje, Marissa Lippert, RD, Eric Beck, Pablo Gallegos, and Kuko. Special thanks to Jen Hoy, who infuses her healing and positive energy into the food and into the recipes she creates. Heartfelt thanks go to my extended team at Finance NYC: Nigel Pierce, Jesse Williamson, and Gonmin Kim for their faith and support. Thank you to other supporters of Mothers & Menus with a shared commitment to empowering new parents, including Julia Beck, Julie Tupler, Carrie Bickner-Zeldman, Manon Chevallerau, Mary Leonard, and Lauren Slayton.

To my own mother, Tami Turel, whose love for children and cooking inspired my own. And to her and my dad, Joe, for setting up "Sababa Camp," the retreat to which my children flocked while mommy typed away. To my in-laws, Anita and Wolf Gurwitz, who always lend a helping hand with love and generosity, and to Serena, our lovely nanny, who mothers my children like her own.

Many thanks go to Dr. David Katz, whose commitment to a healthier nation is surpassed only by his warmth, generosity, and humanity, and to Dr. Laura Riley for her consideration, kindness, and care.

It is with wonderment and earnestness that I gave thanks to my fabulous children Nika, Sophie, and Ethan for their unbelievable patience and for shouting "Go, Mommy, go!" whenever I am nearing a finish line. Special thanks to Nika for her Lemon Cookie recipe, to Ethan for his relentless smiles, and to Sophie for the dime she gave me to "go buy yourself a coffee at Starbucks, Mom."

And finally, my acknowledgment, adoration, amazement, and gratitude go to my husband, Dori, my soul mate, my passion, my partner, and my idol in how he lives his life to the absolute fullest, taking every risk worth taking and staying committed to his vision and our family, holding us all up with his strength. And for always, relentlessly, lovingly pushing me to be the best person I can be. Thank you, Foufi.

Index